MAGICK FROM THE MAT

About the Author

Casey Giovinco (North Carolina) is the Chief Elder of the Gala Witchcraft tradition who has been combining yoga and witchcraft for over twenty years. He has a RYT-200 certification from The Yoga Alliance, teaches yoga, reads tarot, and works as a witch in residence at a holistic center.

USING **YOGA** TO
ENHANCE YOUR **WITCHCRAFT**

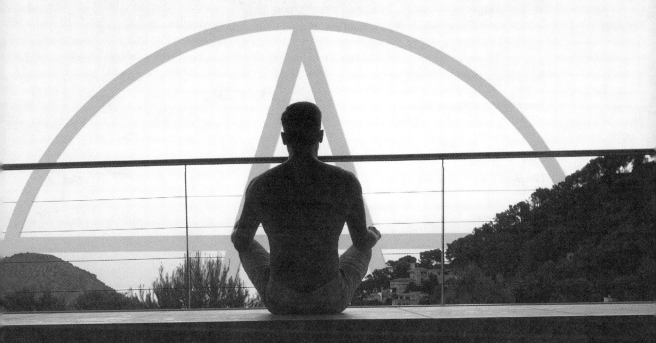

MAGICK FROM THE MAT

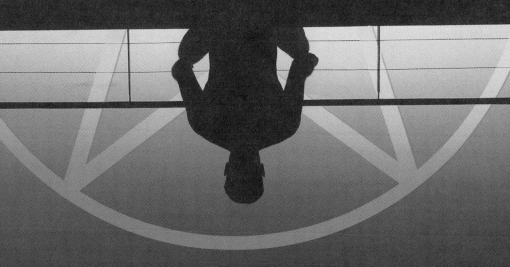

CASEY GIOVINCO

LLEWELLYN PUBLICATIONS
WOODBURY, MINNESOTA

First Edition
First Printing, 2021

Cover design by Shira Atakpu
Interior art by Mary Ann Zapalac

Llewellyn is a registered trademark of Llewellyn Worldwide Ltd.

Library of Congress Cataloging-in-Publication Data
Names: Giovinco, Casey, author.
Title: Magick from the mat : using yoga to enhance your witchcraft / Casey
    Giovinco.
Description: First edition. | Woodbury, Minnesota : Llewellyn Publication,
    2021. | Includes bibliographical references.
Identifiers: LCCN 2021013223 (print) | LCCN 2021013224 (ebook) | ISBN
    9780738765952 | ISBN 9780738766201 (ebook)
Subjects: LCSH: Magic. | Witchcraft. | Yoga.
Classification: LCC BF1623.Y64 G56 2021 (print) | LCC BF1623.Y64 (ebook)
    | DDC 133.4/3—dc23
LC record available at https://lccn.loc.gov/2021013223
LC ebook record available at https://lccn.loc.gov/2021013224

Llewellyn Worldwide Ltd. does not participate in, endorse, or have any authority or responsibility concerning private business transactions between our authors and the public.

All mail addressed to the author is forwarded, but the publisher cannot, unless specifically instructed by the author, give out an address or phone number.

Any internet references contained in this work are current at publication time, but the publisher cannot guarantee that a specific location will continue to be maintained. Please refer to the publisher's website for links to authors' websites and other sources.

Llewellyn Publications
A Division of Llewellyn Worldwide Ltd.
2143 Wooddale Drive
Woodbury, MN 55125-2989
www.llewellyn.com

Printed in the United States of America

To my big sister, who has always had my back. The way you battled cancer during the Covid-19 crisis taught me more about integrity, grace, and strength than you will ever know. I love you.

CONTENTS

EXERCISES

MEDICAL DISCLAIMER

Please consult a medical doctor before you begin any exercise program. While yoga is for everyone and provides amazing health benefits, only you know your own limitations. The techniques and suggestions in this book are not meant as a substitution for medical advice.

FOREWORD

Like a lot of Americans, my own introduction to yoga was as a component of physical fitness. It was an exercise—sort of a fancy way to stretch, and good for when you weren't cut out for team sports. It was offered as an alternative to conventional gym classes at my (admittedly unusual) high school, and it's still a popular way to satisfy the physical fitness requirement at a lot of colleges and universities. Even now, when the New Year rolls around and people start posting about their fitness and weight loss goals, yoga is often front and center. It's touted as a cure-all: tone your body, exercise without strain or the risk of injury, feel sexy, build flexibility, and tune out the stresses of your busy daily life. Come December, my social media feed fills up with ads for local studios, practically always featuring extraordinarily slim, serene-looking models, almost always white, blonde, and fashionably coordinated. For years, I would think, "Good for them. But my body doesn't do that."

When I became seriously involved in witchcraft as a young adult, I was exposed to another yoga entirely. Yoga is everywhere in Pagan, New Age, and other kinds of magical communities, and though the focus isn't usually on physical fitness, it was just as difficult for me to navigate. Wasn't this an Indian tradition? Perhaps even a religion all by itself? I had friends who had grown up in churches that didn't allow members to practice yoga because they saw it as another, conflicting spiritual practice. And here I was, suddenly meeting Pagans who incorporated yoga into their own meditation and ritual practices as though it was a matter of course. But wasn't yoga something separate? Were we just appropriating something out of context?

How confusing! It's a strange thing—yoga is both ubiquitous and mysterious. It's everywhere—both in mundane and magical spaces—and yet it remains widely misunderstood.

I didn't begin to seriously reconsider the practice of yoga from the perspective of witchcraft until I cast a wider net and started learning about the development of contemporary witchcraft—especially Wicca—through the work of Western occultists around the turn of the twentieth century and later. Yoga has a deep and expansive history within its original Hindu contexts, as anyone who explores it readily discovers. What many don't realize, however, is that it also has a rich history among occultists and magicians, long before ever becoming a fitness craze. It is impossible to spend any time at all in occult communities without being exposed to ideas and traditions born in Asia, and then translated through American and European new religious movements, particularly Theosophy. Such traditions often go unsung in popular books, but their influence on contemporary witchcraft of practically any variety you can name cannot be overstated. Indeed, many concepts that we take for granted in Pagan, New Age, and witchcraft communities today—energy healing and balancing, the mind-body connection in matters of health, the emphasis on manifestation—come to us not from our ancient Pagan forebears, but from modern traditions like Theosophy and New Thought. We can thank them (and also critique them) for introducing many Westerners to yoga. We also see yoga when we study ceremonial magic, particularly the works of Aleister Crowley, that most influential of modern occult luminaries. Yoga is simply impossible to avoid, whatever flavor of magic calls to us.

In *Magick from the Mat*, Casey brings all of these worlds together, leading readers on a fascinating tour through history while also detailing how contemporary practitioners—of either yoga or witchcraft—can incorporate their practice of one into the other, thereby deepening them both. This is a massive undertaking, and he handles it with aplomb, doing justice to yoga's rich history outside of Western contexts and advising witches in how they might approach a yoga practice with both respect and confidence. If your objective is to practice yoga for the first time, Casey serves as an experienced, knowledgeable guide who will help you build firm foundations. If you are already firmly rooted in a yoga practice of your own, Casey will teach you to harness what you're already doing and direct it to enrich your life even further through the practice of witchcraft. You don't have to have a particular sort of body or a predetermined level of experience in either yoga or witchcraft to enjoy the wealth of information and encouragement here.

I came to yoga late in life and well into my practice as a witch. It's helped me develop my psychic abilities, build a consistent and meaningful meditation practice, and create the kind of stillness in myself that intense ritual magic work often requires. Aside from all the benefits to my physical and emotional well-being, yoga's allowed me to deepen my work as a magician and witch, in sometimes surprising ways. I now understand why so many recommended it to me when I was younger, and why it was a core element in the practices of so many witches and magicians I've admired throughout my life. On an intellectual level, it's also augmented my understanding of the development of contemporary occultism, and its impact on witchcraft. If you're at all interested in how East and West have overlapped in modern magic, the study of yoga will make those connections apparent, serving as an ideal case study. If your interest is practical, then here are the steps to get you started, from a variety of angles.

Wherever you are on your own path, you could ask for no better guide than Casey Giovinco. An adept and respected witch, as well as a yoga teacher with years of experience in multiple settings, Casey's approach is both practical and profound, with a keen eye toward inclusivity, and the care that spiritual combination and exploration demands. I only wish that my own introduction to yoga had been so aided, but I am grateful to benefit from Casey's work now. We are fortunate indeed.

Thorn Mooney

INTRODUCTION

Imagine...

You inherit the family house from Aunt Fern. To your surprise, the house is fully furnished and move-in ready when you get there. It's almost as if it was waiting for you to come home.

You decide to wander around and explore every nook and cranny of that beautiful old Victorian. Its wraparound porch looks like a splendid place to while away a beautiful summer afternoon or enjoy a midnight margarita while basking in the light of the full moon.

When you walk inside, you find out that your aunt left a veritable treasure trove of antiques and memories. Over the front door is a horseshoe with the ends pointing up toward the ceiling. At the far end of the foyer is a tin star—a pentagram! The fireplace in the living room has a copper cauldron in it, and half-burnt candles are lovingly placed around the hearth. There are even dried herbs hanging from the ceiling in the kitchen. Everything just looks so witchy!

You rush up the two flights of stairs to the attic, which fascinated you to no end as a child. Locked doors have always piqued your curiosity. When you get to that old wooden door, you are delighted to see that it opens for you. You enter the small chamber, and you are struck again by how witchy everything feels. It's just like something out of the late 1990s television series *Charmed*.

In the middle of the room, you see the faint outline of three concentric circles stained into the floorboards, faded by years of sunlight pouring in through a beautiful stained glass window. As you look around, you see countless other magickal-looking items. An antique straw witch's broom sits in the corner. Crystals seem to have been set out purposefully on the windowsill to bathe in the sunbeams. A gilded mirror with inky black glass hangs on one wall, and an old steamer trunk sits in another corner. Its rusty hinges make it difficult to open, but you persist. Inside the trunk, you find a letter addressed to you sitting atop the other contents.

You open the trunk to find a dusty old book. Resting the book on your lap, you flip through its discolored pages until one page in particular catches your eye. It talks about the magick carpet, how to consecrate it, and how to use it once it's prepared. You realize that the dusty old book in your lap must be your aunt's Book of Shadows. You notice a carpet rolled up behind the attic door, and your heart beats a little faster. Do you dare believe that this rug might be the one talked about in the book? If you were to climb on it, where would it take you?

———————

Is it just me, or do all witches dream about things like this?

A generous aunt who leaves you the family house filled with magickal items, a room that was once considered off-limits being opened to you, and ancestral secrets revealed from a rusty old trunk in a dusty old attic—it all feels like the beginning of an Alice Hoffman novel. Doesn't it?

Witches, like magpies, just seem to cobble together the most interesting elements of life, surrounding themselves with magick. However, this talent for acquisition is not just good for decorating romantic Victorian homes. The witch's ability to hunt and peck through other metaphysical systems for the shiny bits of universal occult truth within those systems is unparalleled. Throughout history, witches have borrowed from other sources.

The fact is that witches have had little choice in the matter. Thanks to the Dark Ages in Europe and the brutality of the Christian Church in attempting to eradicate its rivals, witches have had to imitate the inquisitive magpie and persevere through the process of reconstructing tattered magickal and spiritual practices. Though many aspects of witchcraft have survived in part, much of the original material surrounding witchcraft has also been lost to the fires of the Inquisition.

Despite all that was lost to this unholy war on witches, the people who stepped out of the broom closet and into the public eye in the nineteenth and twentieth centuries were not without their resources. By turning to Eastern spiritual traditions and practices like yoga in order to augment what remained of Western occultism, witches (and other occultists) were able to regain some of what was lost in the West with an unbroken line of accumulated wisdom from the East.

Though the concept of combining witchcraft and yoga may seem revolutionary to some people reading this book, the truth is that witchcraft and yoga have been yoked together for well over a century. As early as 1875, the Theosophists were turning to Buddhism and yoga for inspiration.[1] In the early twentieth century, Aleister Crowley compared the classical elements of the West to the practice of yoga. In his *Eight Lectures on Yoga*, Crowley said, "Fire represents the yogi, and water the object of his meditation."[2] Meditation's fluid nature might account for why it is often so hard for new students to gain traction in their practices. Think about that age-old metaphor of trying to hold water in your hand. If you struggle and try to grip the water, you'll displace it, sloshing water this way and that. However, if you cup your hand and hold real still, you'll be able to hold on to the small amount of water that fits within your cupped palm. Meditation, like gripping water, can definitely be an exercise in frustration when starting out. Crowley's comparison seems appropriate.

Meditation is not the only thing that Western occultists have borrowed from the practice of yoga. Even the chakras themselves were not originally part of any Western magickal practice. Those colorful whirling vortexes of energy came directly out of the yoga tradition. Though the Upanishads talk about them as psychic centers and they play a more prominent role in tantra, they are first mentioned in the Vedas. There are

---

1. Debra Diamond, ed., *Yoga: The Art of Transformation* (Washington, DC: Smithsonian Books, 2013), 97.
2. Aleister Crowley, *Eight Lectures on Yoga* (Las Vegas: New Falcon Publications, 1992), 48.

at least twenty-nine direct references to the chakras in the *Rig Veda*.[3] They were added into the witch's concept of energetic anatomy to supplement a still-unknown missing piece of information that was stolen from witches by Christianity in the last two thousand years. There is still so much more wisdom for witches to glean simply by practicing yoga alongside their witchcraft.

History of Yoga

According to Mark Stephens in his book *Teaching Yoga*, "What we know of the origins and development of yoga comes to us from a variety of sources, including ancient texts, oral transmission through certain yogic or spiritual lineages, iconography, dances, and songs... the earliest known writings on yoga are found in ancient Hindu spiritual texts known as the Vedas."[4]

Some accounts of the Vedas date them as being nearly twenty-five hundred to three thousand years old. Though they are often thought to be the original written source material for yoga, the Vedas mostly discuss meditation through the practice of mantras. The actual practice that we identify as *yoga* didn't get thoroughly explained until the Upanishads were written down in the first millennium BCE. The *Bhagavad Gita*, being the most famous of the Upanishads, helps the reader find inner peace and bliss by connecting with Divinity.

It is in the Upanishads where the Hindu religious philosophy that influenced much of yoga was written down. Within these later texts, we find a discussion of the universal spirit, Brahman, and a distinct individual soul, Atman, discussed in depth. The Upanishads also talk about subtle body anatomy and the life force energy, prana, that permeates all things. Considering how much of this material has worked its way into modern witchcraft almost verbatim, it might not be too far a stretch to say that these texts could be seen to be just as sacred to modern witches as they are to Hinduism.

---

3. "Chakras within the Vedas: Stopping Scholarly Distortion of Vedic Texts," *Hindu Human Rights Worldwide*, July 13, 2020, https://www.hinduhumanrights.info/chakras-within-the-vedas-stopping-scholarly-distortion-of-vedic-teachings/.

4. Mark Stephens, *Teaching Yoga: Essential Foundations and Techniques* (Berkeley, CA: North Atlantic Books, 2010), 1–2.

As foundational to understanding the metaphysical wisdom of yoga as the Vedas and the Upanishads undoubtedly are, many modern yoga students and teachers have never read them. That is not the case with Patanjali's *Yoga Sutras*, however. The yoga sutras—or just sutras, as they are sometimes called—are nearly ubiquitous in the modern Western yoga community. The sutras are a brief, but powerful, 196 aphorisms, which were written down sometime between 500 and 400 BCE. Some of the Upanishads were written after Patanjali put pen to paper, and his work certainly influenced them. In this text, Patanjali asks, "What is yoga?" His answer is both elegant and powerful. The famous sage discusses how practicing yoga can calm the mind and reveal the nature of one's True Self through the blissful state of samadhi.

Another World Tree

Yoga is often compared to a tree. As a witch, I have always appreciated this metaphor, because it, more than anything else, seems to unite the two distinct paths so elegantly. The World Tree is often associated with various branches of witchcraft, and many witches have magickal practices that include making pacts with trees.

Yoga is seen to have roots, a trunk, branches, blossoms, and fruit, just like a tree. In his commentary on Patanjali's *Yoga Sutras*, B. K. S. Iyengar expounds on this beautiful imagery. He talks about how the eight branches of yoga could be seen as a tree.[5] Here is a paraphrasing of his metaphor:

1. Yama, or ethical behavior, is like the roots of the tree.

2. Niyama, or personal observances, function as the trunk, providing stability and structure to a yoga practice.

3. Asanas, or the physical postures, are the branches, which move and flow with the breeze.

4. Pratyahara, or internal focus, is the bark that provides a barrier between the internal workings of the tree and the external elements.

5. Dharana, or focused internal concentration, is represented by the tree's sap.

---

5. B. K. S. Iyengar, *Light on the Yoga Sutras of Patanjali* (United Kingdom: HarperCollins UK, 2002).

6. Pranayama, or the breath, is represented by the leaves of the tree.

7. Dhyana, or becoming one in body, breath, and mind, is seen as the flower of whole consciousness.

8. Samadhi, or pure bliss, is represented by the fruit.

To add witchcraft into this beautiful metaphor and combine the two paths in a unique way that still honors the individual beauty of each, it might be appropriate for witches who wish to add yoga into their magickal practices to think of witchcraft as the primordial soil that nurtures the roots of this wonderful tree. Though this association may seem a bit odd given that I just finished discussing how modern witchcraft has been augmented by yogic wisdom, it shouldn't trip the reader up too much.

The history of witchcraft as an archetypal concept is just as ancient as yoga. Stonehenge, a site sacred to many modern witches because of its possible connection to the Druids and its role as a possible sacred space in historic Pagan spiritual practices, is from the same period that the Vedas were written down in. It was built around 3000 BCE. There are also remnants of shrines, tools, and cave paintings that strongly suggest some practice similar to what we might call witchcraft existed as far back in history as 50,000 BCE.

How to Use This Book

As the title of this book suggests, yoga can be used to enhance witchcraft, but witchcraft can also be used to enhance a yoga practice as well. However true those statements are, this book is not meant to unite the two distinct paths into something new, making "yoga witches" or something else of the sort. That would only disrespect the integrity of both systems, which are whole and beautiful in their own right.

Rather, this book seeks to explain universal occult truths by comparing the similarities between two distinct traditions. Yoga and witchcraft are more like complementary sister traditions that can enhance each other. By adding witchcraft to yoga, yogis progress more quickly on their paths. By adding yoga to witchcraft, witches develop their psychic powers more efficiently, which, ultimately, deepens their spiritual experiences in witchcraft.

While reading through the pages of this book, consider reading each chapter in its entirety before doing the exercises within it. That way the full scope of the connection between yoga and witchcraft is understood and you can better apply that knowledge to the exercises. In this way, you will progress much more quickly and be able to adapt the material to your own personal magickal practice. Blessed be and namaste.

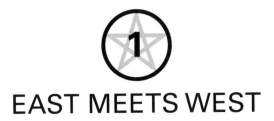

EAST MEETS WEST

Most people in the West today think of yoga as being exclusively about exercise. It's not. As Iyengar's tree metaphor shows, the asanas are just one small part of the overarching tradition that is yoga. The occult aspects of this ancient spiritual practice actually dwarf the physical sequences.

The benefits of yoga for solitary witches cannot be overstated. Yoga actually provides the solitary practitioner with the same depth and breadth of psychic training, which was, until very recently, reserved almost exclusively for coven-based, initiatory witchcraft. Coven-based witches in initiatory traditions have the benefit of learning from the successes and failures of the witches who have come before them in their lineage. They can streamline their progress along the Path of the Wise (another name for witchcraft) and develop their psychic potential so much more quickly and easily because of that initiatory connection. Unfortunately, solitary witches rarely have that same benefit.

I should know. My own witchcraft practice has been both solitary and coven-based at different points in my life, and yoga has been a great boon to me during both phases of my own magickal development. As a young adult, I spent much of my time in bookstores thumbing through the books on witchcraft and the occult, trying to decide which one to take home. Generally, I made my decision based on countless hours of deliberation, comparing the author's personality to the usefulness of the spells or rituals, which were detailed in those wonderful books.

Unfortunately, once the initial excitement of a new purchase had subsided, I often found myself disappointed in my choice. Even though I religiously followed the directions in those books, it always felt like my spells just didn't work. I blamed myself. I thought it must have been my fault. Clearly, it couldn't be the author's fault. After all, they were witch enough to get a book contract. That had to count for something.

Then one day during a yoga class, I stumbled upon the solution to my magickal problem. Though I was diligent in following the directions in the books, I wasn't concentrating enough on my goal when it came to casting the spells. This revelation happened completely by accident. At the end of the class, during savasana, or corpse pose, I was lying flat on my yoga mat with my eyes closed in a meditative state. My mind drifted to thoughts of a spell from one of those books that I wanted to cast later that night.

For the entire savasana, I visualized what it would be like for that spell to work. I imagined my life after successfully casting it. I focused on that desired outcome as if it had already come to pass, and I maintained that focus to the exclusion of everything else. In fact, I was so deeply entrenched in my thoughts during that savasana that I remained in the trance state long after that class had ended. The teacher had to politely nudge me after everyone else had packed up just so the next class could come into the studio.

To my surprise, that particular spell worked. I got exactly what I wanted, exactly as I had visualized it during my savasana. Looking back on it now, that shouldn't have surprised me. That deep level of concentration is at the heart of all successful magick. However, back then, this accidental discovery was earth-shattering. After that success, I started a personal practice of doing yoga before every spell or ritual, and, to my delight, my magick started to work more often than not.

It wasn't until I joined the coven where I was formally initiated into witchcraft that I learned the reason why adding yoga to my witchcraft practice generated success. During my training for initiation, my teacher spent a great deal of time focusing on the importance of concentration and visualization. As a devout yoga student by that time, I immediately recognized the similarities between the meditation exercises he gave me and my own experiences with my savasana practice.

Imagine my surprise when I found out that it wasn't just me. The realization that yoga had actually influenced the overarching tradition of witchcraft was mind-blowing.

Yoking Yoga & Witchcraft

Though adding yoga into your witchcraft practice may seem like a novel concept, it is not new. According to Kurt Leland, a modern Theosophist, the period between 1880 and 1990 shows a drastic and organic growth of a unique interpretation of the chakras. The evolution of the Western chakra system started with the works of Helena P. Blavatsky in 1880 and fully materialized with Shirley MacLaine's appearance on *The Tonight Show*.[6]

Western occultists have been using yoga to augment the Western Occult Mystery Traditions, including witchcraft, for over a century. Things like the chakras, much of our modern understanding of occult anatomy, and even the label *New Age*—which some modern energy workers apply to their magickal and spiritual practices—all worked their way into witchcraft through the Theosophical study of yoga and Hindu texts.

In some cases, the Theosophists deviated dramatically in their interpretations. In other cases, they stuck very closely to the original source material. Whether those alterations were necessary to educate Western minds or those changes could be seen as cultural misappropriation remains a heated topic for debate. On the one hand, the Theosophical interpretations of yogic philosophy cause confusion. On the other hand, many Westerners owe a debt of gratitude to the Theosophists for the mass spiritual awakening of the twentieth century, which came out of their work.[7]

Just considering the chakra system alone, most of what Westerners know and love about the chakras comes directly out of Theosophy. The color correspondences, the elemental associations, even the connections to the nervous system that most people

---

6. Kurt Leland, "The Rainbow Body: How the Western Chakra System Came to Be," *Quest*, Spring 2017, 25–29.

7. "New Age Movement: Religious Movement," *Encyclopedia Britannica*, accessed July 13, 2020, https://www.britannica.com/topic/New-Age-movement.

associate with the chakras—these are all additions that were never part of the traditional Hindu theology.

Yoga Defined

In the *Rig Veda*, we learn that *yoga* can mean *to yoke* or *to make one*.[8] However, the word actually has many meanings. According to *Yoga Journal*, "The Sanskrit word *yoga* has several translations and can be interpreted in many ways. It comes from the root *yug* and originally meant 'to hitch up,' as in attaching horses to a vehicle. Another definition was 'to put to active and purposeful use.' Still other translations are 'yoke, join, or concentrate.'"[9] When the word *yoga* is translated as *to yoke* or *to join*, the translator is prioritizing the science of uniting a human spirit to Divinity or helping the person reconnect with the True Self. This is the meaning that has achieved prominence within Western translations.

Though less common, the other translations cannot be ignored entirely, because they reveal more of the occult and esoteric wisdom inherent in the practice of yoga. For example, by acknowledging the essential element of concentration, as the *Yoga Journal* writer did, a deeper understanding of the process of union can be realized. The *Yoga Journal* writer is pulling this translation from Vyasa's commentary on Patanjali's *Yoga Sutras*. In that commentary, Vyasa says, "Yoga is Samadhi or Perfect Concentration."[10] It is this less common translation of the word *yoga* that is most in line with the witch's path, because it reveals that yoga, like witchcraft, is ecstatic in nature.

Yoga & Psychic Powers

Before we discuss how yoga can benefit the witch's psychic and magickal development, however, we should talk about a point of disagreement between the two traditions. For many people who practice yoga, the conscious pursuit of psychic development

---

8. Stephens, *Teaching Yoga*, 2.

9. "A Beginner's Guide to the History of Yoga," *Yoga Journal*, accessed May 13, 2020, https://www.yogajournal.com/yoga-101/the-roots-of-yoga.

10. "Vyasa Comments on Yoga: Section 1 (Aphorisms 1-13)," *Sanskrit & Trika Shaivism*, accessed May 13, 2020, https://www.sanskrit-trikashaivism.com/en/vyasa-comments-on-patanjali-yoga-sutras-I-1-13/632#Vyaasa11.

is seen to be a frivolous distraction. Some practitioners feel very strongly against the topic.

I remember one particularly heated discussion on psychic powers during a yoga teacher training that I took a few years back. The instructor brought up the topic of the *siddhis* (the word used in yoga philosophy for psychic powers), and you could practically see the battle lines being drawn. When the traditional perspective held by most yoga practitioners in the West was given by the instructor, one woman said that she flat-out disagreed. She was very open about her own psychic abilities, and she didn't appreciate being told that her gifts were distractions from spiritual enlightenment. To be honest, I couldn't fault her there. A few of the students in the class were really harsh in their response to her. Though there was an attempt to return order, the teacher eventually had to shut the conversation down and dismiss the class for the day. I have also seen similar things happen in online groups when someone asks about the siddhis or psychic powers in general.

This aversion comes from a long line of sages who talk about yoga, but in the West, most people learn about the yoga philosophy regarding psychic powers through Patanjali's *Yoga Sutras*. For Patanjali, the universe is dualistic. It is composed of both Spirit and matter. After spending some time detailing the dualistic nature of the universe, Patanjali cautions the reader against the concerted effort to develop psychic powers.

For Patanjali, concentration is a mystical experience meant to unite the practitioner with Spirit. Everything outside of that ultimate goal is seen as a distraction. As in aphorism III, 38, Patanjali tells us that the psychic gifts, which have a tendency to develop naturally from yoga and the trance state, present obstacles to spiritual growth.[11]

Magick & Mysticism

Initially, it was very hard for me to reconcile Patanjali's *Yoga Sutras* and their supposed philosophy against psychic powers. My spiritual beliefs and my personal experiences seemed to counter his wisdom. My own spiritual awakening as a witch was transcendent, and I attributed a great deal of that transcendence to my intense focus on psychic development. It made me feel closer to my God and Goddess, and it gave me a connection to Spirit that I had completely lacked before.

---

11. Mukunda Stiles, ed., *Yoga Sutras of Patanjali* (San Francisco: Weiser Books, 2002), 41 (III, 38).

It was years before I was able to resolve this cognitive dissidence within myself. As I studied the sutras and I learned more about the process of enlightenment within Hindu theology, it became easier to see the fine distinctions that Patanjali was making. He was not actually against psychic powers. By his own admission, psychic powers are a natural potential outcome of a regular yoga practice. That this is so can be seen in Patanjali's description of the three transformations of the mind and the psychic powers that develop out of them.

All three of these mental transformations or shifts have their root in the harmonious integration of contemplation, meditation, and being absorbed in Spirit. Patanjali refers to this harmonious integration as *samyama*.[12] In witchcraft, this same process is often referred to as *ecstasy*. During the first mental shift, the attention turns inward.[13] During the second shift, all distraction disappears and a single-pointed focus occurs.[14] Finally, all thoughts cease entirely within the mind during the third transformation.[15] When this final shift happens, the psychic powers begin to develop naturally.[16]

Rather than renouncing psychic powers, Patanjali merely argued against actively seeking to develop psychic powers. If you look at aphorism III, 38 again, Patanjali merely says that they are "impediments" or distractions from the ultimate goal, which is "being absorbed in Spirit." It is actually the duality of consciousness between the Self and the mind that stands at the very heart of the sage's criticism of psychic development, since psychic development strengthens the mind and binds the Self or Spirit to the material world.

When discussing the development of psychic powers, though, it is important to realize that Patanjali is not just talking about the development of things like telepathy, prophecy, or other magickal abilities. He warns against conscious association with all aspects of what he calls "the worldly mind" in aphorism III, 38. This includes things that many of the other students who attacked my classmate in that yoga teacher training would prize as necessary to normal, everyday human interactions.

---

12. Stiles, *Yoga Sutras*, 32 (III, 4).

13. Stiles, *Yoga Sutras*, 33 (III, 9).

14. Stiles, *Yoga Sutras*, 33 (III, 11).

15. Stiles, *Yoga Sutras*, 34 (III, 12).

16. Stiles, *Yoga Sutras*, 35 (III, 16).

According to this philosophy, any ability the mind has to interact with the external world is suspect. That includes reason, logic, feeling, external perception, empathy, or any other faculty that may currently be studied by science. The rational mind and the Higher Self are absolutely distinct from each other. The Higher Self exists above the mundane experiences of daily existence. It is our illusory connection with the worldly ego that distracts us from recognizing our true selves.[17]

Patanjali hits this point home very early on in his *Sutras*. In the first chapter, he tells us that the Self gets wrapped up in the thoughts of the lucid mind and loses sight of the fact that it is actually the subject experiencing those thoughts.[18] If you want to see a real-world example of this, look at method actors who struggle to regain their own identities after particularly intense roles, and you'll understand Patanjali's point.

He also points out that the obstacles to recognition of the Transcendental Self are qualities that we typically associate with the mental landscape of human consciousness. Even normal processes of the rational mind are viewed to be problematic for Patanjali. Things like perception, understanding, imagination, sleep, and memory all distract us from our true selves just as much as psychic abilities do.[19]

The witch, however, takes a more pragmatic view. Whereas yoga philosophy depicts the mind as just another layer of matter that is meant to be overcome on one's path to enlightenment, the witch who approaches witchcraft as a spirituality sees the material nature of the mind as simply another tool to be utilized in pursuit of unification with Deity. The spiritual witch recognizes that there is an important metaphysical reason for "worldly minds." There are karmic lessons through the process of reincarnation that simply cannot be learned without those minds.

A foundational concept within many branches of witchcraft is that the witch has one foot in the realm of the living and the other foot in the realm of Spirit. This philosophy insists that the witch straddle the hedge and navigate both the mundane and spiritual worlds adeptly,[20] learning to be a fully functional member of society and a spiri-

---

17. Stiles, *Yoga Sutras*, 40 (III, 36).

18. Stiles, *Yoga Sutras*, 2–3 (I, 4).

19. Stiles, *Yoga Sutras*, 2 (I, 2).

20. Arin Murphy-Hiscock, *The Way of the Hedge Witch* (Massachusetts: Provenance Press, 2009), vii–viii.

tual adept at the same time. By maintaining this balance, the witch progresses lifetime after lifetime through the process of reincarnation toward an eventual and well-earned enlightenment.

Therefore, when witchcraft is treated as a religion, it is always a spirituality of the world. After all, that is part of what people mean when they say that witchcraft is a nature religion. Witches embrace the natural world and garner wisdom from that interaction. Being a rather practical approach to spirituality in that way, the practice of witchcraft encourages and prepares witches to meet their basic material needs before they approach the more esoteric elements of the Craft. From the witches' perspective then, it is certainly understandable why people might look down on spending countless hours a day navel-gazing if meditators also struggle to pay their rent, put food on the table for their families, or meet life's other necessities.

The witch's answer?

Develop the psychic powers of the mind and use them effectively to cast spells or perform magick rituals to get ahead in this world. The psychic powers of the mind are essential to success in this endeavor. However, after comfort and success have been attained, the wise witch then turns to the Great Work of identifying the True Self, the Higher Self—or what Patanjali called the Transcendental Self—just as the yogi does.

In truth, the philosophical approaches of yoga and witchcraft are not that far apart on the topic of psychic powers. Patanjali encourages readers to live in accordance with nature's cycles in order to be elevated from the cycle of reincarnation.[21] The witch simply sees the material nature of the mind as a natural resource that must be tapped wisely in order to achieve the reunification with Spirit that Patanjali advocates. Franz Bardon probably said it best in the introduction to his book *Initiation into Hermetics* when he said, "there is no difference between magic and mysticism,"[22] and the spiritual witch wholeheartedly agrees.

---

21. Stiles, *Yoga Sutras*, 47 (IV, 2).

22. Franz Bardon, *Initiation into Hermetics* (Salt Lake City, UT: Merkur Publishing, Inc.: 2001), 17.

Three Mental Shifts

If you would like to witness Patanjali's description of the mental transitions from the *Yoga Sutras* for yourself, seat yourself comfortably on the floor or in a straight-backed chair. If you're on the floor and it's comfortable, cross your legs in the standard meditation position. In yoga, this is called *lotus pose*. If you're seated in a straight-backed chair, place your feet on the floor and rest your palms on your thighs. Start with five minutes for each phase of the mental shift. Then progress from there. The progressions are enumerated in simple, easy-to-follow steps below:

1. In the beginning, it is important to merely observe your thoughts. Watch them. Discern a pattern. Get to know your own thought process intimately instead of just taking it for granted. Refrain from judging your thoughts. Just observe your thoughts. Allow your mind to wander. Witness the distraction as a dispassionate observer. When you have succeeded at this endeavor for the predetermined time, add one minute to your next practice session. Do this until you have achieved a focused, concentrated thought for ten uninterrupted minutes.

2. After you have succeeded at focusing your attention on simply observing your thoughts, change strategy and begin to control them. During this phase of your meditation practice, try to focus your mind on one thought. For the sake of simplicity, start out by contemplating a piece of fruit. Take an apple, an orange, a lemon (whatever appeals to you). Study it with your eyes open. Then at the beginning of your meditation practice, close your eyes and re-create that piece of fruit in your mind's eye. Hold your thoughts on that one agenda alone. Staunchly refuse to allow other thoughts to intrude upon your meditation. When you have succeeded at this endeavor for the predetermined time, add one minute to your next practice session. Do this until you have achieved a focused, concentrated thought for ten uninterrupted minutes.

3. Once you have mastered that exercise, start over at five minutes again, but this time empty your mind entirely. Think of absolutely nothing; just be present in the moment. Allow yourself to drift in this state of bliss and contentment without errant thoughts, feelings, or impulses influencing your mental, emo-

tional, or physical state. Maintain this equilibrium for five minutes. Then, when you've achieved success at emptying your mind for the predetermined time, increase your next practice session by one minute. Repeat this process until you've achieved ten minutes again.

This process should take you roughly a month.

The Hermetic Approach

It is only a matter of perspective that separates yoga and witchcraft philosophies, not belief. As with all conflict, the resolution of this apparent disagreement rests in clarifying the concept of truth being debated. In *The Kybalion*, we find out that there is a paradox surrounding the nature of the universe. Looked at from an absolute viewpoint, the universe is simply a mental creation of Spirit, a figment of the divine imagination or an illusion. This is the perspective espoused in texts on yoga. However, looked at through a relative lens, the universe is actually very real indeed. This means that at all times the universe is both illusion and reality. It really just depends on how someone chooses to look at it in the moment.

From the absolute viewpoint, only the eternal and unchanging is real. Within this perspective, the only thing that truly qualifies as eternal and unchanging is Spirit or Deity. Everything else is illusion. The concept of the dreamer and the dream is often used to describe this theory.

However, the absolute perspective is only half the story. It's the story from the divine perspective. It says nothing of humanity's perspective within the dream. Though it is easy to write a dream off as illusion upon waking up, the events are all too real while the dreamer dreams. The knowledge of the dream's illusory nature does little to help the dreamer negate the emotional investment in the Dreamtime, even upon waking up. That is the situation a human spirit faces during each incarnation.

The relative viewpoint addresses this perspective by erecting the actor's fourth wall and makes the dreamscape as real as waking reality while the dream is in progress. By buying into the context of the dream, the overarching story line can be played out to its natural conclusion and the dreamer wakes up with new insight.

Whereas the yogi wants to avoid the distraction of the dream and get back to waking reality as quickly as possible, the witch recognizes the need to be able to balance between the two modes of consciousness—dreaming and waking, illusion and reality, material and subtle. For the witch, the distraction of the dream that is life has its uses within the waking world of Spirit. Time spent in the incarnated dreamscape can be just as insightful as waking up from a revelatory night's slumber after spending days or weeks grappling with a major life decision.

The I & the Me

Within the dualistic universe that he establishes in his philosophy, Patanjali describes three eternal, coexistent principles: Deity, the Self, and matter.[23] Consciousness becomes dualistic as a spirit descends into matter. While interacting with the physical realm, consciousness alternates between pleasure and pain. In fact, in most texts on yoga, this duality of pleasure and pain is the very hallmark of the embodied human mind. Only by transcending the confines of that mind and embracing our true nature as the Transcendental Self can we get above the fray.

In aphorism I, 24 in his *Yoga Sutras*, Patanjali talks about how an individual's Transcendental Self is untouched by karma or its effects.[24] In fact, the unassailable nature of the Transcendental Self when it comes to karma is the reason that people focus so much on transcending the mind through meditation during a yoga practice. By quieting the famous monkey mind of the mundane ego, we begin to hear the call of the Self and, thereby, begin to minimize suffering. All the things that happen to us (even our thoughts and feelings) in this lifetime do not harm who we truly are.

The witch also recognizes these three eternal, coexistent principles. Oddly enough, the roots of the witch's version of this particular wisdom surround the ivory tower of Western academic philosophy. William James in his book *The Principles of Psychology* (1890) understood what René Descartes failed to grasp: we are not the thinking thing.[25] Rather, we are the thing that experiences the process of thinking. We are the

---

23. Patanjali, *Patanjali's Yoga Sutras*, trans. M. A. Rama Prasada (New York: AMS Press, Inc., 1974), i.

24. Stiles, *Yoga Sutras*, 8 (I, 24).

25. René Descartes, *Discourse on Method* (Auckland: SMK Books, 2009).

thing that experiences the thoughts themselves. In aphorism II, 20, Patanjali tells us that the Higher Self is an experiencing thing. He calls it "the seer" and ascribes only consciousness to it. While it directs thoughts and concepts, the mind's operations do not impact it.[26] In *The Principles of Psychology*, James distinguished two understandings of the Self. He identified the Self as Me and the Self as I. The Self as Me is an object of the experiences an individual has. The Self as Me is defined by those life experiences. Whereas the Self as I is the subject having the experience in question.[27] I like to think of these two aspects of consciousness as the role an actor plays (Me) and the actor playing the role (I).

James's understanding of consciousness works its way into witchcraft through *The Kybalion*, which tells us that "a man thinks of his Self (in its aspect of 'Me') as being composed of certain feelings, tastes, likes, dislikes, habits, peculiar ties, characteristics, etc., all of which go to make up his personality, or the 'Self' known to himself and others."[28] Basically we find that this version of the Self is made up of the experiences had by the person in question. *The Kybalion* is equally as revealing about the I of James's philosophy. As a person's consciousness evolves and becomes more spiritually aware, the I, the actual Self, becomes easier to see. Associations with the physical body and the pull of its influence are less dramatic, and the individual is able to disentangle from the trappings of the mundane ego and its various mental and emotional states. "After this laying-aside process has been performed, the student will find himself in conscious possession of a 'Self' which may be considered in its 'I' and 'Me' dual aspects."[29] This process of laying-aside reveals the True Self of Patanjali's *Yoga Sutras* or what modern witches might refer to as the Higher Self.

The Siddhis

If we start with comparing Charles G. Leland's *Aradia or the Gospel of the Witches* to chapter 3 of Patanjali's *Yoga Sutras*, we see that both traditions talk about psychic

---

26. Stiles, *Yoga Sutras*, 21 (II, 20).

27. William James, *The Principles of Psychology* (Mineola: Dover Publications, 1950).

28. Philip Deslippe, ed., *The Kybalion: The Definitive Edition* (New York: Jeremy P. Tarcher/Penguin Group, 2011), 169.

29. Deslippe, *The Kybalion*, 171.

powers being founded in love. In *Aradia*, Leland tells us that Aradia can gratify those who conjure her by granting them with success in love.[30] While the witch focuses on love being the reason for developing these powers, Patanjali suggests that love is also the key to accessing them. Both aphorism III, 24, and aphorism I, 33, talk about love in one form or another. Aphorism 33 of chapter 1 talks about bringing joy to others and relieving them of their burdens.[31] Though he doesn't come right out and say it explicitly, Patanjali is talking about an occult principle that witches know all too well. Love is the highest vibration. In order to access the full scope of any power, you must align yourself with its highest frequency: love.

This is not some platitude meant to minimize other emotions. Love comes in many varieties. It can be soft and gentle, but it can also be cold and aloof. A mother's tough love is equally as necessary for the successful raising of her children as the tender loving care she gives when she tucks them into bed at night. Being higher than all the other vibrations, love operates above them all, and can often accomplish what nothing else can.

As for the psychic powers themselves, they are also talked about in similar ways. In some places they are actually talked about identically. Leland details eleven different powers claimed by the witches who follow Aradia. Let's look at them one by one next to Patanjali's corresponding aphorisms.

Leland tells us that a witch has the ability to "bless or curse with power friends or enemies."[32] One common way that a witch blesses friends and curses enemies is through the use of the elements. The same mastery can be achieved through a regular yoga practice. Patanjali tells us that "by the practice of samyama on the various states of the elements—gross, intrinsic, subtle, all pervasive—and seeking to know their abundant purposes, one gains mastery over the elements."[33]

According to Leland, a witch has the ability to converse with spirits.[34] Two different aphorisms in Patanjali's *Yoga Sutras* ascribe the same power to yoga practitioners,

30. Clayton W. Leadbetter, ed., *Aradia or the Gospel of the Witches* (Franklin Lakes, NJ: New Page Books, 2003), 35.

31. Stiles, *Yoga Sutras*, 10 (I, 33).

32. Leadbetter, *Aradia*, 35.

33. Stiles, *Yoga Sutras*, 43 (III, 45).

34. Leadbetter, *Aradia*, 35.

though he uses a different vocabulary to talk about these abilities. He says, "From this discrimination spiritual perceptions are born in all the senses"[35] and "By the practice of samyama on the interrelationship of hearing and the element of ether as space, one experiences the omnipresence of divine hearing."[36] Together, these sound very similar to spirit communication to me.

Leland details two ways that witches can become wealthy. They have the ability to find hidden treasures in ancient ruins or through necromancy and mediumship, conjuring the spirits of priests who died leaving treasure.[37] Patanjali tells us that yoga practitioners can acquire wealth through spiritual means as well.[38] As to what "wealth" entails in either of these traditions, this is a topic for another day. For now, it is enough to show that they are both talking about the same thing in similar ways.

Both the witch and the yoga practitioner are said to be able to divine. Leland tells us that the witch has the power to divine with cards and to know the secrets of the hand.[39] Patanjali encourages us to meditate on the quality, character, and condition of the mind in order to gain knowledge of the past and future.[40]

The power to cure disease is ascribed to both witches and yoga practitioners alike. Leland claims it outright.[41] Patanjali suggests that meditation on the navel chakra will bring the ability to heal the body and bring it back to proper functioning.[42] The following aphorism, which talks about controlling the metabolism, further hints at the power to heal through conscious control of the body.

---

35. Stiles, *Yoga Sutras*, 40 (III, 37).

36. Stiles, *Yoga Sutras*, 42 (III, 41).

37. Leadbetter, *Aradia*, 35.

38. Stiles, *Yoga Sutras*, 43 (III, 46).

39. Leadbetter, *Aradia*, 35.

40. Stiles, *Yoga Sutras*, 35 (III, 16).

41. Leadbetter, *Aradia*, 35.

42. Stiles, *Yoga Sutras*, 38 (III, 31).

The witch has the power to make those who are ugly beautiful.[43] So does the yoga practitioner. In aphorism III, 47, Patanjali tells us that the yogi has the ability to perfect the body in various ways. One of the perfections he mentions outright is beauty.[44]

Finally, Leland and Patanjali both agree that the witch and the yoga practitioner share powers over the animal kingdom. Leland tells us that the witch has the power to talk to beasts.[45] Patanjali, on the other hand, claims that words themselves are what cause confusion. By meditating on the spirit of the communication, one is given clarity regarding the speech of all living beings. Presumably, that includes animals as well.[46] Though he talks about verbal speech a great deal here, presumably the fact that Patanjali chose the phrase "all living beings" instead of saying something like "humanity" indicates that he meant to include animals, plants, or any other living being within the scope of this power.

Though both authors present powers and abilities that the other leaves untouched, the similarities listed should make a good case for adding yoga to the witch's psychic development. The witch and the yoga practitioner are working along similar and compatible energetic currents, and yoga can be immensely useful in helping witches to further develop their psychic powers.

Meditation for Healing

Before you begin this exercise, determine something you would like to heal in yourself. This can be an upset emotional state or a physical condition that has been causing you to feel unwell. Create an image in your mind that symbolizes success in this endeavor. If it's an emotional dis-ease, maybe you see yourself smiling, surrounded by friends who love you. If it's a physical condition like a broken leg, maybe you see yourself strong and healthy, dancing all night long.

Once you have determined what you will heal during this meditation, take up the lotus position or sit in a straight-backed chair with your feet placed firmly on the floor.

---

43. Leadbetter, *Aradia*, 35.

44. Stiles, *Yoga Sutras*, 43 (III, 47).

45. Leadbetter, *Aradia*, 35.

46. Stiles, *Yoga Sutras*, 35 (III, 17).

You will be repeating the second phase of the previous exercise. Simply hold your mental focus on one thought for five solid minutes without allowing other thoughts to creep into your mind. This time, your thought will be one of healing.

Close your eyes, and focus on your breath. Breathe in and out through the nose. Take a few deep belly breaths. As you breathe in, feel your stomach inflate like a balloon. As you exhale, imagine yourself pulling your belly button in until it touches your spine. Expel all the stale air. Do this about five times before you turn your mind toward your navel's psychic center. While you can certainly attach various correspondences to this meditation, they are unnecessary. All you need to do is focus your awareness on the navel, right around the region of your belly button.

After you have established a rhythm that works easily for you, pull your image of you healthy and happy up in your mind. Hold that image firmly before your mind's eye, and focus on it and nothing else for the duration of your meditation. When you lose your focus, open your eyes. Your body has processed all the healing energy it can at that time. Repeat this meditation as often as you like until your emotional or physical health has improved to your satisfaction.

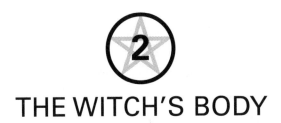

THE WITCH'S BODY

Your body is a temple.

The words are so easy to say. If only applying the philosophy to daily life were that easy! Unfortunately, it's so much easier to talk about treating the body right than it is to actually do it. A common complaint is that good food just tastes so damn bad. Another issue is that working out feels like torture to some people. As a personal trainer and a yoga teacher, I've heard it all. Believe me.

Trying to live by the your-body-is-a-temple philosophy and maintain the conveniences of modern life can be endlessly frustrating. People are overworked and underpaid. Even if people want to eat right and exercise more often, they face the daunting task of just trying to find the time. While society talks about a forty-hour work week, the reality is that most people routinely work fifty hours a week or more. Spread out over five days, that means that most people spend roughly ten hours a day at work. Even worse, too large a percentage of society has to work on the weekends or has a second job just to make ends meet. There's actually very little time left to plan and cook a good quality meal each night or to routinely hit the gym.

A Healthy Mind in a Healthy Body

Though the wisdom about treating the body as a temple has become commonplace and rather universal in our colloquial language, few people know where it comes from. The original source of this now ubiquitous concept actually has its roots in Biblical soil. When the Apostle Paul confronts Christians at the church in Corinth, he asks, "Do you not know that your bodies are temples of the Holy Spirit, who is in you, whom you have received from God?"[47] Though Paul is arguing against what he perceives to be sexual immorality in this quote and though most of the witches I know would strongly disagree with his opinion, it's hard to deny that there is wisdom in treating the body in healthy ways.

Fortunately, the Christian Bible is not the only source we have to turn to for guidance on this topic. Providing for the physical health of the body is a part of most spiritual practices. Hebrew has its Kosher Laws. The Hindu faith is intimately connected to the practices of Ayurveda and yoga. I have long believed that witches might have had something similar connected to witchcraft before the Inquisition. If you look at common books on wortcunning or herbalism, you can see how this might be true.

Thich Nhat Hanh said, "Keeping your body healthy is an expression of gratitude to the whole cosmos—the trees, the clouds, everything."[48] Juvenal, the Roman poet, said, "Mens sana in corpore sano," which is usually translated as "a healthy mind in a healthy body."[49] Even the Buddha said, "To keep the body in good health is a duty ... otherwise we shall not be able to keep the mind strong and clear."

The Forgotten Witch's Tool

For witches who desire to be successful in the Craft, it is absolutely essential that some care and attention be put into improving or maintaining their physical health. This may sound judgy or unsympathetic to many people, but it's not. This level of care has nothing to do with fitting into some idealized representation of beauty. It's also

---

47. I Corinthians 6:19–20.

48. Thich Nhat Hanh, *Touching Peace* (California: Parallax Press, 2009), 89.

49. Sybil Leek, *The Complete Art of Witchcraft* (New York: Signet, 1971), 110–11.

not about fat-shaming or criticizing people for circumstances that are beyond their control.

The level of care and attention that witches choose to pay to their bodies is relative. For some people, it might just be eliminating one thing, like soda, from their diet. For others, their plan of care may include simply going for a walk around the block. Still others might actually go all out and join a gym or yoga studio. The point is not that you have to do any one specific thing. Rather, the point is that you just have to embrace the idea of paying some more attention to the maintenance and well-running of your physical body. Let that be whatever it is for you, and don't let anyone judge you for your efforts. That also means don't judge yourself!

As Sybil Leek, who was billed as "Britain's most famous witch" by the BBC,[50] pointed out, "One of our tenets, then, is the Tenet of the Balanced Life."[51] She goes on to say that witches should "consider all things that refuse to allow the body to function in the way it was designed to act."[52] She includes things like illness, hygiene, proper nourishment, and physical abuse within the scope of this consideration. Starting with any of these areas of life in some small way is all that is necessary to get the mojo going.

Another reason that witches need to take care of the physical body is because it directly impacts the success of a witch's ability to raise and manipulate energy. The physical body isn't just a temple for witches. It is actually a magickal tool, like the athame, the wand, or the cauldron.

Gerald Gardner tells us that "witches are taught and believe that the power resides within their bodies which they can release in various ways, the simplest being dancing round in a circle, singing or shouting, to induce a frenzy; this power they believe exudes from their bodies…"[53] I have always had a theory that the power that Gardner mentions exuding from the witch's body is what Allan Kardec, the famous medium and author, was referring to when he talked about the ectoplasm of manifesting mediums.

---

50. "Sybil Leek—The South's White Witch," *BBC Inside Out*, accessed June 22, 2020, http://www.bbc.co.uk/insideout/south/series1/sybil-leek.shtml.

51. Leek, *The Complete Art*, 110.

52. Leek, *The Complete Art*, 111.

53. Gerald B. Gardner, *Witchcraft Today* (New York: Citadel Press, 1970), 20.

This energetic release hints at one of the more well-kept secrets surrounding the witch's Circle. Many witches will tell you that the Circle is a boundary, and so it is. However, it is also a container. It assists in accumulating and holding the energy as it pours off the witch's body. Once the Circle is saturated with this energy, the witch "programs" it with a specific intention and then directs it toward the target of the ritual or spell.

Generating & Seeing the Witch's Energy

If you should wish to see the witch's power exuding from your own body as Gardner described, this simple exercise will help you do just that. Make sure that you practice this exercise on an empty stomach. Once you eat a heavy meal, the body begins conserving its energies for the physical process of digestion. It helps to be able to see this energy if you are naked, but that's not necessary. You can always choose to wear clothing that leaves your arms and legs exposed and achieve success with this exercise.

1. Dim the lights.

2. Dance around in a circle for five to ten minutes, singing your favorite song as you whip yourself up into a frenzy.

3. Stop and stand facing a white wall.

4. Hold your hand out at arm's length in front of you so that the white wall serves as background. Gaze at the edges of your hand, and observe the fine white mist that surrounds the fingers.

You have just witnessed the witch's power emanating off your body. If you still doubt the body's role in raising this energy, simply repeat the exercise again at another time. However, on your second experiment, leave out the dancing and singing. Just dim the lights and gaze at your hand against the background of a white wall. Notice the differences for yourself.

Mind-Body Connection

The physical body is not the only body that witches need to consider in the process of leading a balanced life. Most spiritual systems talk about people having several bodies—a physical body and various other subtle bodies. A common metaphor for talking about this concept is the Russian nesting dolls. Both yoga and witchcraft philosophies have similar versions of this subtle anatomy, and a comparison of these individual systems might prove useful here.

The Five Sheaths

As with the Russian dolls, yoga's version of subtle anatomy approaches the physical body as the largest doll, the outer sheath, and works inward to the core of the person's being—the embodied soul. The theory dates back to the Taittiriya Upanishad, which was most likely composed in the sixth century BCE.

That sacred text details three bodies or *shariras* and five sheaths or *koshas* in order to map the inner journey of yoga. The three bodies are *sthula* or the physical body, *sukshma* or the subtle body, and *karana* or the causal body. The five sheaths are *annamaya* or food, *pranamaya* or energy, *manomaya* or mind, *vijnanamaya* or intellect, and *anandamaya* or bliss.[54]

As Mark Stephens says, "Hatha yoga is a means for becoming consciously aware of this interwoven fabric of existence, connecting the physical and subtle bodies, bringing awareness more and more to a place of blissful being."[55] By practicing yoga and becoming more consciously aware of the various subtle bodies described in the Upanishads, witches can be more effective at finding a balance between the mind, body, and spirit that works for them in their individual lives.

Theosophy & the Seven Principles

The understanding of subtle anatomy that is taught in my lineage of witchcraft traces its roots back through the Theosophists and yoga to the Ancient Wisdom Religion. The Theosophists refer to this theory as *The Seven Principles of Man* or *The Septenary*

---

54. Stephens, *Teaching Yoga*, 48.

55. Ibid.

Nature of Man.[56] Like the Five Sheath theory from yoga, it is appropriate to conceptualize the Theosophical theory through the lens of the Russian nesting dolls, ascribing the largest of the dolls to the physical body.

The first principle or aspect considered in the Theosophical theory is the physical body. It is the vehicle that contains all the others during a person's incarnated lifetime. The vital body, or what is called *pranamaya* in yoga philosophy, immediately follows next in line as the second principle. The astral or etheric body is catalogued as the third of these principles. In addition to serving as a vehicle of travel for the consciousness during out-of-body experiences, it also serves as a template of sorts, holding the pattern for the energetic makeup of the dense physical form. The fourth body in the *lower quaternary* is the desire body. This principle is the root of our passions, impulses, instincts, and drives. It is often called the *animal soul* or the *lower manas* in some Theosophical texts.

In addition to the animal soul or the lower manas, there is also a higher, thinking mind, which the Theosophists call the *higher manas, manas* just being another word for mind. In her book *The Seven Principles of Man*, Annie Besant says, "I will ask the reader to regard Manas as Thinker rather than as mind, because the word *Thinker* suggests someone who thinks, i.e., an individual, an entity."[57] This principle is also referred to as the Ego. It is the Self as I of both James and the Hermetists discussed earlier.

The sixth principle is referred to as the Buddhi or Spiritual Self, which serves as the link between the Ego and Deity. When it is combined with the upper manas, it is also seen as the Divine Ego. Without being yoked to the upper manas, the Buddhi aspect serves merely as a vehicle for the seventh and final principle, the Atma or Atman, which is also referred to as the *divine ray of the Universal Self,* the *Higher Self,* or *Deity.*

Conclusion

Witches who wish to succeed more easily with their own psychic and magickal development could do no better than to turn to yoga for guidance and inspiration. There

---

56. H. P. Blavatsky, *The Key To Theosophy* (New Zealand: Pantianos Classics, 1889), 53.

57. Annie Besant, *The Seven Principles of Man* (London: The Theosophical Publishing Society, 1909), 25.

are many points of similarities between the two traditions that will enhance the witch's spiritual practice and practical training. However, there are also gaps in witchcraft because of the Western history of witch hunts. Yoga can help fill those gaps.

For example, by understanding the Five Sheath theory, which inspired the modern holistic mind-body-spirit philosophy we all know so well,[58] it becomes easier for witches to transcend insecurities and doubts that they may have in any one problematic area of their lives. In Jnana-style yoga, there are meditations specifically designed to help yoga practitioners dissolve their association with each sheath—something witches have been decidedly silent about in publicly available material.

58. Stephens, *Teaching Yoga*, 48.

GUIDELINES FOR A
MAGICKAL YOGA PRACTICE

Both yoga and witchcraft help practitioners *know thyself.* That is actually the primary aim of yoga and one of the main reasons why it is so useful for witches who wish to develop their psychic powers. The physical postures that make a regular yoga class are seen as tools that help yoga students better connect with, understand, and transmute their base Egos into their True Selves. In a sense, the physical postures are really just the beginning of yoga. They were designed specifically to get the physical body out of the way so that meditation could happen without interruption.

Once the awareness of this True Self begins to take root in the consciousness, the meditative practice of yoga helps students balance the opposites within themselves. Positive and negative, physical and spiritual, hot and cold—these are all opposites balanced within a yoga practice. Even the word *Hatha*, which is associated with most of the varieties of yoga practiced in the West, can be translated as *sun and moon*, indicating the essential component of balance within a yoga practice.

Another reason why a regular physical yoga practice can benefit the witch is that it is preparing the body to be an efficient vehicle for prana, which is often translated as *breath* or *life-giving force*. Witches refer to this same concept by many names. Some witches have borrowed the words *prana*, *akasha*, and *kundalini* from yoga. Other witches simply call it *ether*, *energy*, *magick*, and many other names.

The Basics

Yoga is more than just stretching and getting into various poses. This truth becomes even more relevant when yoga is added to a witch's psychic and magickal training. There is actually an energetic component to each physical pose that must be experienced in order to actually be "doing yoga."

In every yoga pose, there is a dynamic interplay of expansion and contraction. Again, the balance of polar opposites comes into play, and through balancing these opposites, power is generated. As you inhale, you expand your lungs along with the rest of your torso. As you hold your breath for a brief moment in the stasis phase of the pose, you begin to generate heat within the body. This physical fact has energetic implications that are essential to the successful practice of witchcraft. By generating heat within the physical body, the witch succeeds at lighting up the astral body. After all, heat and light are both just different aspects of the fire element.[59] As you exhale and release the energy that you have been holding within, you cool the body down and produce a feeling of relaxation and calm. In that still moment after you have exhaled the last of the breath before you inhale again, you create a space for introspection to take place.

However, the breath is not the only place where this interplay of opposites happens. For every pose, there is a counter-pose that balances it. For example, a forward fold is often balanced by a backbend in a yoga class. You have periods of dynamic flow where you move through a sequence of poses very quickly, having one movement align with one breath. The fast-paced flow sequences are often followed by periods of

---

59. Bardon, *Initiation into Hermetics*, 30.

static holds where several very slow, deep breaths elapse as you hold one specific pose, deepening the experience as the mind's eye turns inward on itself.

Types of Poses

A yoga class will generally include a variety of poses to balance the body and stabilize the mind. It will also touch on active and passive postures to produce heat or cool the students off. Within Hermetic philosophy, this combination of active and passive polarity is often talked about as electric and magnetic, so if witches were to apply the Western occult vocabulary to developing a personal magickal yoga practice, they would talk about balancing their bodies and minds with electric (active) and magnetic (passive) poses. This could be done in line with a specific intention before a spell or ritual—i.e., to increase a witch's ability to project power out or to accumulate power within—or merely as a workout to maintain the health of the body.

Here is a brief introduction to eight different types of poses that will help prepare the body to achieve a specific intention. With these eight types of poses, the witch can design a personal yoga practice for any magickal intent.

Standing Poses

Where witchcraft has the concept of grounding and centering, yoga has the **standing poses**. With your feet firmly rooted into the earth, these poses provide both strength and stability. Some basic poses in this category include the following:

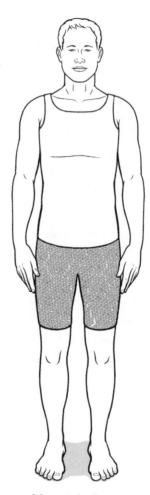

Mountain Pose

- mountain (tadasana)

- garland pose (malasana)

- warrior I (virabhadrasana I)

- warrior II (virabhadrasana II)

Balance Poses

Some of the standing poses are actually considered **balance poses**. Because of their difficulty, balance poses, whether standing or not, do so many things. On a physical level alone, they relieve stress, reduce anxiety, build core strength, and develop full-body awareness. On a magickal level, these poses help develop the witch's will by improving memory, concentration, and focus. Some basic poses in this category include the following:

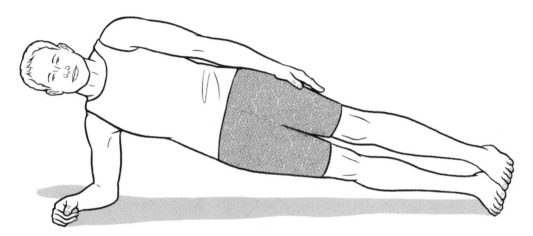

Side Plank Pose

- side plank (vasisthasana)

- plank pose (utthita chaturanga dandasana)

- warrior III (virabhadrasana III)

- half moon pose (ardha chandrasana)

- crow pose (bakasana)

- scale pose (tolasana)

Inversions

Inversions help conquer fear and overcome adversity. Most people shy away from these poses, because they are perceived to be difficult, requiring a combination of balance, flexibility, and strength. However, the truth is that there are a variety of levels of intensity when it comes to inversions. Some are, indeed, quite challenging, but others can actually be peaceful and relaxing once the fear factor is removed. By changing our orientation to the world around us, these poses give us a new perspective on life. They also increase circulation and stimulate the brain. As a result, mental clarity is achieved. These poses also help witches see beyond the illusion of the current situation, and for witches who work with the witch's pyramid, inversions help with the *to dare* portion of the pyramid. Some basic poses in this category include the following:

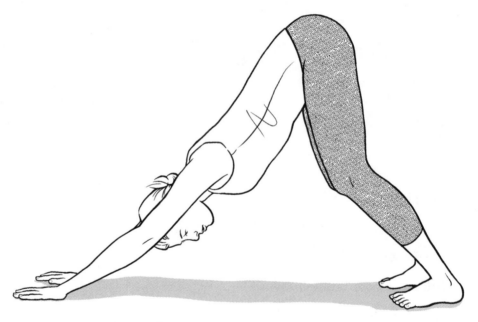

Downward-Facing Dog Pose

- downward-facing dog (adho mukha svanasana)

- legs up the wall pose (viparita karani)

- supported shoulderstand (salamba sarvangasana)

- plow pose (halasana)

Twists & Binding Poses

Twists and **binding poses** are excellent at purifying both the body and the mind. On a physical level, these poses aid in digestion, stimulate the liver and kidneys, and help evacuate the bowels, which assists in removing toxins and waste from the body. On the mental plane, twists and binding poses work to purge the mind of thoughts that aren't appropriate to the present moment. In some branches of witchcraft, the scourge serves this same purpose. That's why the scourge is part of the purification process to get ready for certain rituals in witchcraft. In addition to their purifying benefits, twists also have the characteristic of lengthening the spine and energizing the body. Some basic poses in this category include the following:

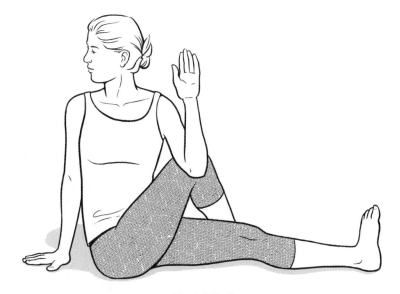

Marichi's Pose

- noose pose (pasasana)

- pose dedicated to the Sage Marichi I (marichyasana I)

- Marichi's pose (marichyasana III)

- half lord of the fishes pose (ardha matsyendrasana)

- revolved side angle pose (parivrtta parsvakonasana)

- revolved triangle pose (parivrtta trikonasana)

Seated Poses

Aside from improving flexibility and stability, **seated poses** help open up both the body and the mind. Static seated poses show up a lot in meditation practices and pranayama. This is one of the reasons that most people identify the simple seated pose, often called easy pose or sukhasana, as the standard position for meditation. Seated poses that are combined with forward folds or twists provide the extra benefit of stability—being connected to the earth—as the main action is happening.

The symbolism of this can be used to great purpose by a cunning witch. For example, perhaps you need to purify yourself of fear. You might decide to take up a seated position on the ground and contemplate your fear. Scan your body with your mind's eye, and find out where that fear resides. After finding the fear, you might choose to add in the element of the twist and imagine that you are wringing out a wet rag as you release the fear from where it has been lodged inside of you.

Some basic poses in this category include the following:

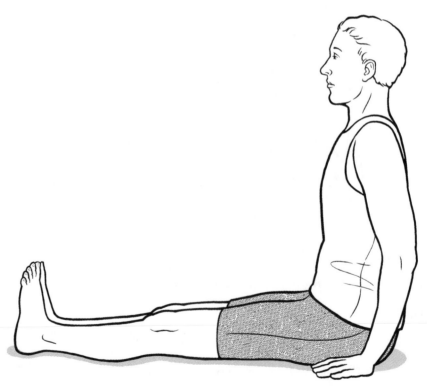

Staff Pose

- staff pose (dandasana)

- seated forward bend (paschimottanasana)

- lotus pose (padmasana)

- hero pose (virasana)

- easy pose (sukhasana)

Forward Folds

Similar to inversions, the **forward folds** are excellent for reducing all forms of stress, including anxiety, depression, and fatigue. They calm the mind and soothe the nervous system. In addition to their many wonderful physical benefits, forward folds also have the wonderful quality of restoring energy levels, so when a witch is feeling depleted or just in need of a quick energy boost, these poses will do the trick. Another benefit is that they do not require a great deal of flexibility. All that is required is that the head is below the heart. This can be done sitting down or standing up. Some basic poses in this category include the following:

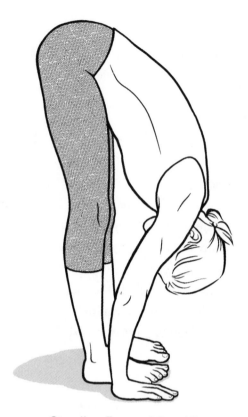

Standing Forward Bend Pose

- big toe pose (padangusthasana)

- child's pose (balasana)

- downward-facing dog (adho mukha svanasana)

- standing forward bend (uttanasana)

- standing half forward bend (ardha uttanasana)

Chest Openers

At the heart of the matter, **chest openers** help with being more compassionate, releasing emotional pain, and, ultimately, embracing more love in general. By the nature of the fact that lifting the chest also arches the back, these poses strengthen and lengthen the spine. They are also useful in opening up the shoulders. Truthfully, by focusing on the chest openers, you can heal the entire upper body. It's quite beautiful how that works. Some basic poses in this category include the following:

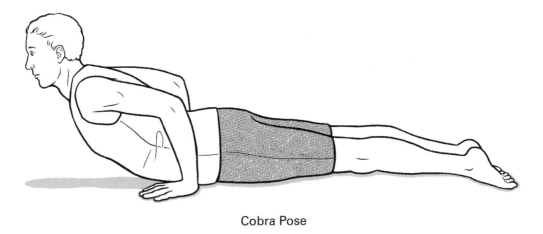

Cobra Pose

- camel pose (ustrasana)

- cobra pose (bhujangasana)

- cow pose (bitilasana)

- locust pose (salabhasana)

- wheel pose (urdhva dhanurasana)

Hip Openers

You might think that the heart chakra and chest openers are the place to focus on when you're dealing with traumatic experiences and pent-up negative emotions, but more often than not, those issues are stored energetically in the hips. **Hip openers** create the space for an energetic release to happen within the root chakra, and through that release, hip openers help people regain control when the emotional pressure becomes too much. Over time, negative emotions begin to hold less sway over us when we make hip openers a regular part of our yoga practice. Situations that used to be traumatic or merely stressful are felt less intensely. Some basic poses in this category include the following:

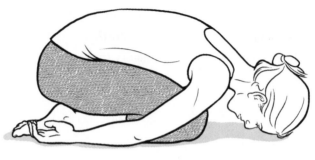

Child's Pose

- bound angle pose (baddha konasana)

- reclining bound angle pose (supta baddha konasana)

- child's pose (balasana)

Contraindications

When we talk about *countraindications* in yoga, we are talking about physical conditions that would make practicing a particular pose or series of poses unwise in a specific moment in time. The conditions that cause contraindications are not always severe. In fact, some are actually quite commonplace. Some are chronic, and should be a regular consideration for your continued yoga practice, and others are fleeting or cyclical. What you should take away from this section is the awareness that you need to pay attention to your own body, that some days you may need to treat your body with some extra tender love and care. If you have any doubts at all about a particular pose, please go talk to a local yoga teacher in person, or if the concern is severe enough, you should consult a qualified medical professional.

Contraindications range from something as simple as dealing with a headache to something as severe as high blood pressure or heart problems and everywhere in-between. This section does not have an exhaustive list, and it should not take the place of appropriate medical attention for your particular situation. However, here is a brief rundown of some common contraindications you might be dealing with in your own life.

Asthma

If you are suffering from asthma, you want to avoid poses that close off the airways or compress the abdomen. Poses like head-to-kenn forward bend or plow fit into this category. You also want to be careful of extremely strenuous poses that work the abdominals, like boat, as they will exasperate your condition. That said, yoga is extremely useful when dealing with asthma, and you should not be afraid to practice as long as you listen to your body. The benefits of yoga for asthma sufferers are immeasurable. Yoga increases airflow while clearing the lungs and building lung capacity. A regular yoga practice also soothes the body and reduces stress, which has been correlated with an increase in asthma attacks.

Back Injury

If you have a severe back injury, please consult a qualified medical professional before starting a yoga practice. If your back injury is relatively minor, be especially careful with heart openers and forward folds. Back injuries are not something to take lightly. Even the most minor aches and pains can be indicative of larger problems. If you have any doubts at all, it is better to be safe than sorry. Consult the appropriate qualified medical professional.

Neck Injury

Neck injuries are another severe condition that should not be taken lightly. If you have any neck problems whatsoever, even ones you consider to be minor, you should consider getting them checked out before practicing yoga.

Heart Problems

It sounds like common sense, but it is important that it be said: if you have heart problems, consult your physician before doing yoga. Avoid the more strenuous poses, especially inversions, like handstand or supported headstand. Even some of the pranayama (breathing) exercises can become problematic if your condition is severe enough. If your doctor gives you permission to practice yoga, start slow. Be gentle with yourself, and consider hiring a yoga teacher to help you with a few one-on-one private sessions in the beginning of your yoga journey.

High & Low Blood Pressure

Both high and low blood pressure are equally problematic. For both conditions, it is really important to listen to your body and recognize the signs of a problem before it's too late. For high blood pressure, pay attention to when your breathing becomes rapid or when you are unconsciously holding your breath. If you do nothing else for your high blood pressure in a yoga class, avoid inversions. For low blood pressure, pay attention to your vision and your equilibrium. If you experience darkness creeping in along the edges of your vision or you feel dizzy, stop. Don't push beyond it. It may be a sign that you need to pay attention to something that is happening within your body. Avoid balance poses and any asanas that have you changing the elevation of your head very rapidly. For example, coming up from a forward fold back into mountain pose can often give people with hypotension some problems.

Menstruation & Pregnancy

In addition to all the other contraindications, most women have two extra conditions that they need to be mindful of when practicing yoga: menstruation and pregnancy. During menstruation and pregnancy, it is advisable for women to avoid twists, inversions, abdominal strengthening exercises, like boat, or pulling the belly button into the spine in any extreme way. While pregnant, it is also advisable not to compress the belly against the ground in prone position (where you are facing the floor). It is also worth noting that you should not engage in any form of breath retention while pregnant as this practice can deprive the fetus of necessary blood flow.

––––––––––

Let me repeat that this is by no means an exhaustive list of all the possible contraindications that you might experience. To list all of them would exhaust this book and several more. If you have any doubts about your own health or your ability to safely begin a yoga practice of your own, please consult a qualified medical professional regarding your unique situation.

Proper Alignment & the Bandhas

Whenever I teach a yoga class, I always find myself repeating the same five things over and over again, regardless of what pose we happen to be practicing in class that day. "Tuck your tailbone. Pull your belly button in toward your spine. Lift your chest. Pull your shoulders back and down away from your ears, and breathe." These five cues are the very essences of good form and proper alignment in a yoga class. If you remember them in every pose, you'll be more likely to do the pose correctly with or without the guidance of a yoga teacher observing you.

Remember:

- Tuck your tailbone.

- Pull your belly button in toward your spine.

- Lift your chest.

- Pull your shoulders back and down away from your ears.

- Breathe.

You'll notice that I always start with the tailbone and work my way up to the shoulders. Then I remind the students to breathe. Ideally people would be consciously breathing throughout the entire yoga class, but you'd be surprised just how often people need to be reminded to breathe. Many people hold their breath when they concentrate, and they just "forget" to breathe until their body's natural mechanisms kick in and force the process.

In general, you should balance yourself from the ground up. If you're performing a standing pose, start with your feet and work your way up. "Build the base" and then stack the rest of the form on top of that stable base. If you're sitting or lying down, start with the root chakra or pelvic floor muscles and work your way up through the relevant points on the body.

Another benefit to beginning with the tailbone and working up the spine is that it helps remind people about the bandhas, which are so important in both the physical and the energetic practices of yoga. They become even more important when witches practice yoga. Whether they know it or not, the bandhas are what help witches raise energy within our bodies. We always talk about raising the kundalini or "feeling the power rise" in various styles of magick and energy work, but most witches never stop to think about what is actually happening within their bodies as they raise the energy. The bandhas can help shed some light on Gardner's quote from the last chapter about the power residing within the witch's body.

The word *bandhas* translates as *to bind or tie back*. They are body locks in Hatha yoga, and they function very similarly to the scourge in Wicca. When we engage the bandhas, we are actually tightening or flexing specific muscle groups in order to "lock down" a part of our physical body, manipulate the blood flow, and contain energy within the flexed area. On the energetic plane, they operate very much like the binding cords and body position that are used with the scourge. On the physical plane though, the bandhas help us develop and maintain proper alignment.

There are three commonly acknowledged bandhas: mula bandha, uddiyana bandha, and jalandhara bandha. Variations of the mula and uddiyanna bandhas are actively involved with producing proper alignment in most yoga poses. The jalandhara bandha is used less often for physical alignment purposes, but should always be done with the full version of the uddiyana bandha.

Mula Bandha

The mula bandha can also be thought of as a *root lock*, because it begins by tightening the muscles of the perineum, or the pelvic floor. A simplified version of this exercise is what the modern medical community refers to as a *kegel*. If you have ever tried to stop urinating midflow, you have identified and worked with the root lock. Simply call that memory to mind and seek to replicate it again. If you struggle to relive the experience, try cutting off your flow of urine next time you go to the bathroom and pay attention to the sensations that produce success.

Activating the Mula Bandha

If you would like to try activating the mula bandha at other times than when nature calls, try the following exercise when your bladder is empty. When you attempt to activate the mula bandha in a yoga or witchcraft practice, also make sure you have an empty bladder. Not only will the experience be less effective on a physical level, but a full bladder could distract you from paying attention to the subtle energies and even compromise the success of a spell or ritual.

You can sit on a chair, lie down on a bed or on the floor, or sit on the floor in a comfortable position. For this exercise, it doesn't matter. Some yoga teachers will advise that their students try to develop control over this bandha in hero pose, because it provides the best positioning for the tailbone, and the perineum is suspended in midair between the calves of the legs with the heels pressed against the glutes. However, this pose can be hard on the knees for some people, and it is not essential to getting the idea. Sit in a way that is comfortable for your body and that will allow you to focus on the exercise itself.

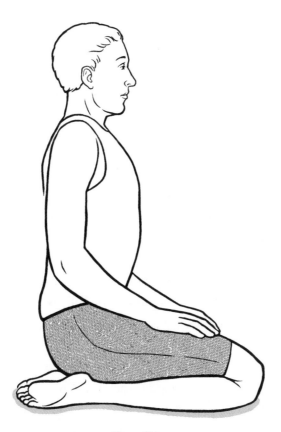

Hero Pose

Should you wish to do this exercise in the recommended hero pose, here are some simple instructions to get you into it. Start on your hands and knees in tabletop position. Now slowly sit back on your heels. Make sure that the tops of your feet are lying flat against the floor. Don't curl your toes under. Try to bring your thighs together, unless that causes pain. Then adjust accordingly until you are comfortable. Rest your hands on your lap, and straighten your back, and elongate the neck, letting your head float gently above your shoulders. This is basically the entire pose.

Once you have found your comfortable position and you are ready to begin, perform a standard kegel, or imagine stopping urinating midstream. On the first day, tighten the pelvic floor muscles for five seconds. Then release. Take a five second break, and then repeat the process four or five more times before ending the session. Slowly build up until you can hold the tension for ten seconds at a time. As I said, the kegel is a simplified version of the mula bandha. If you want to learn the full version, seek out the guidance of an experienced yoga teacher so that you ensure you are doing it correctly and not risking unnecessary injury.

Uddiyana Bandha

The second body lock is referred to as *uddiyana bandha* in yoga. The word *uddiyana* translates as *up* or *upward* in English, and that is exactly what this body lock is doing. It's pulling the belly button back and up toward the spine. In my yoga classes, I simplify this as "pull the belly button in toward the spine" because this is the easiest way for people to gain an understanding of what is happening with this particular bandha. However, this is just another simplified version. It is not the full lock. Like the kegel and the mula bandha, simply pulling the belly button in tight is like riding a bike with the training wheels on. It helps you get the idea without exposing you to unnecessary risk.

There are some important considerations to take into account before attempting this bandha. Whereas the mula bandha required an empty bladder, the uddiyana bandha requires an empty stomach. Don't try to do this when you are full. The results may be unpleasant. Unlike the mula bandha, most teachers will teach uddiyana in a standing position until the students become proficient at it. Should you wish to practice this bandha beyond the simplified version that I use in most of my classes, here are some simple guidelines to help you navigate the practice. If you struggle with performing this exercise, you feel uncomfortable in any way, or you get light-headed while doing it, please talk to a qualified medical professional and then, with their permission, consult a local yoga teacher in your area who can help you perform this particular exercise.

Activating the Uddiyana Bandha

If you want to give it a whirl in the privacy of your own home, here are the basic steps that most yoga teachers teach their classes:

1. Begin by bending your knees slightly.

2. Round your torso and place your hands on your thighs. Avoid pressing on the knees.

3. Inhale deeply through the nose.

4. Fill your lungs completely. You'll know you're doing this if your belly begins to expand like a balloon.

5. Exhale forcefully through your nose, contracting your abdominal muscles as you do so. Imagine that you are pulling your belly button back as close to your spine as possible. It should feel as if your belly button is moving back and upward underneath the rib cage. You want to expel as much of the air that you just inhaled as possible.

6. Relax your abdominal muscles.

7. Expand your rib cage as if you were going to take another breath in, but don't actually breathe. You are just puffing up your torso here.

8. Hold for a moment.

9. Repeat the process.

Jalandhara Bandha

Jala is usually translated as *net*, which makes sense for what this bandha or lock is doing on an energetic level. It catches energy like a net catches fish. This bandha actually does seem to work like a net. The suffix *-dhara* is often translated as *support*. So, by combining the words *jalandhara bandha*, we get a net that supports the lock, and that's sort of what it does. This bandha actually supports the other two locks.

As a witch, I like to think of this bandha as the cork or stopper on the alchemist's crucible. I have often found that when I want to raise energy for a particular spell, I can engage the mula and jalandhara bandhas and run energy through the energy centers between the two points. This technique builds the power within my own body before releasing it to charge a particular working.

Activating the Jalandhara Bandha

To perform this bandha, sit in a comfortable position. Pull your shoulders back and down so that you lift your chest. Many beginning yoga students simply lower the chin a little bit, which is okay. It will produce a mild version of this bandha, but the full version requires you to lift your sternum in order to meet your lowered chin. This is where the alchemist's crucible metaphor becomes useful. Think of the dual action of lifting the sternum and lowering the chin as corking the flask. You want to press these two points together and seal off the opening of that imaginary flask.

After you get the hang of the jalandhara bandha on its own, try adding in the uddiyana bandha. Exhale all the air out of your lungs, as discussed in the uddiyana exercise. Start by holding the two bandhas for five seconds. Inhale normally as you release both bandhas. Then wait at least five seconds before repeating the process four or five more times before ending the session. Build up your practice sessions to do five to ten rounds, holding your breath for ten seconds and having ten seconds of rest between each repetition.

Going back to the discussion on contraindications, do not attempt to do the uddiyana or jalandhara bandhas if you have hypo- or hypertension. These are part of a breath control practice called *pranayama*, and they should only be approached by people who are healthy enough for regular physical activity. If you have doubts about your own ability to do these exercises safely, err on the side of caution until you can talk to a qualified medical professional.

Props

As Westerners, we have conditioned ourselves to be competitive. No matter how many times yoga teachers tell their classes that they shouldn't compare themselves to anyone else, no matter how frequently these teachers cue their students to turn their attention inward, Western yoga students tend to struggle with a tendency to compete or to compare themselves unfavorably against other people in a yoga class. "Am I doing the pose right?" "Jimmy is so flexible. I'll never get my knees to touch the ground like he does." "My savasana doesn't look like that!" People will beat themselves up over the simplest things, and though it's unfortunate, it's a necessary fact that yoga teachers in the West have to address. Most beginning yoga students are just going to spend a great deal of time comparing themselves against the other people in a class.

It's a dreadful habit that we all really ought to do away with.

Speaking from personal experience, the very best place to do away with this tendency to compete and compare is in the use of props. When you start out with yoga, do yourself a favor and use every prop you can get your hands on. I know that it might be a blow to your ego initially. It certainly was to mine, but if you take my advice here, if you are gentle with yourself and you use the props so that your alignment is correct, you will notice progress so much faster than if you try to "muscle through" the difficult beginning stages of a new yoga practice.

Some common props that you can use during a yoga class include the following:

- The wall—a wall is one of the most useful props available to you. Nearly everywhere that you will choose to do yoga, you will have access to some sort of wall. If you are ever in doubt about whether or not you can sustain yourself in a pose, whether that be a balance pose, an inversion, a forward fold, or something else, move over to a wall and begin practicing the pose using the wall as support.

- A chair—another free and quite useful prop that we all have around our houses is the basic straight-backed chair. In fact, this prop is so useful that there are even chair yoga classes available at fitness centers all over the world.

- Blanket—even a standard, run-of-the-mill blanket, like the kind you curl up with to watch a movie on the couch, can make an excellent prop during yoga practice. It can be used to cover your body during meditation sessions, but it can also serve as a bolster to prop up or support various parts of your body for many seated and supine postures.

- Bolsters—these work exactly the same as a rolled up blanket. They come in various sizes to accommodate different body types.

- Blocks—the block can be made of wood or foam. Most of them these days are foam. What's important is the size of the block and that you are able to grip its edges easily. You generally want a block to come about halfway up your calf when it is set vertically on the floor. When it's laid flat, you want it to be just above your ankles. Most blocks are standard sizes these days, so I wouldn't worry too much about the fit, unless you are extremely tall or short. Blocks are most useful when your hamstrings or hips are tight.

- Straps—last, but certainly not least, are the straps. These are the best prop a new yoga student can invest in. They allow you to deepen your stretch while maintaining proper alignment in all variations of yoga poses. They're useful standing, sitting, prone, or supine. Straps are ideal for stretching the hamstrings, but I have seen some clever yoga teachers and students repurpose these props in the most fascinating ways. There's really no limit to what you can do with a proper strap.

Preparing for Practice

When you get ready to start your own yoga practice, whether in a class with a yoga teacher or at home on your own, there are a few things you need to keep in mind.

Remember: yoga is not a competitive sport. Please do not compare yourself to anyone else. Your body is unique, so it requires unique treatment. If you listen to your body, you are much less likely to injure yourself. Be mindful, stay present in the moment, and listen to your body.

When you are attempting to get into a pose, seek both stability and comfort in equal measure. You can certainly push yourself to go deeper. That's how progress is made, but pay attention to that moment when tension gives way to pain. Always pull back to a comfortable depth before the pain sets in.

Start slow, and be steady in your practice. Give yourself the freedom to progress naturally over time. You should never force the process or go beyond the point of work into the realm of struggle and strain.

Finally, breathe. It's important.

Trying It Out

It is just unfortunate that most discussions on alignment and body mechanics do not include the energetic components talked about in this chapter. My hope is that, by engaging the bandhas when you practice the physical postures, you will remember that you are actually still working with energy. Yoga, especially yoga done with the bandhas in place, is not just a physical exercise. It's magickal training, just like any of the psychic development exercises you might be asked to do in standard Wiccan or witchcraft 101 books.

For this exercise, stand in mountain pose. It was described on page 36. Again, do not do this exercise if you have a medical condition that is contraindicated for the uddiyana and/or jalandhara bandhas.

1. Observe your breath for a moment.

2. After observing the breath's natural rhythm, begin to take control of it. Consciously slow the breath down so that you are taking about eight seconds on the inhale, pausing for four seconds, and exhaling for eight seconds. Feel each breath going deeper and deeper into the lungs. As it does so, your belly should expand like a balloon. When the belly fills completely, the rib cage should begin expanding out.

3. Once you have control over the breath, add in the mula bandha. Squeeze the pelvic floor muscles. Then begin the next cycle of breathing. Hold the pelvic floor tight through the entire length of the breath. As you inhale, visualize yourself taking in universal energy. See it traveling down to the root chakra, which becomes more and more vibrant as you do so. As you pause between inhale and exhale, see the root chakra begin to expand and the energy begin to rise up. Then exhale, emptying your mind of all thoughts.

4. Do the same thing again, but this time on the exhalation, engage the uddiyana bandha as well. Bend your knees slightly, place your hands on your thighs, and round your back as you exhale all the air out of your lungs, pulling your belly button back and upward toward your spine as you do so.

5. Hold the stasis between breaths for a brief moment. Then release the bandhas. Stand up and give yourself a moment before starting the next round.

6. Engage the mula bandha again before starting this third round. Repeat the visualization. Then repeat step 4. As you hold the stasis between breaths on this round, move your hands to your hip bones. Without breathing in, straighten your spine, raising your torso upright and lifting the chest. If you can visualize the energy rising up from the root during this movement, do so. If not, just get the hang of the motion. You'll eventually be able to combine them.

7. Repeat step 6, but this time add in the jalandhara bandha into the mix. As you straighten your spine and raise your chest in uddiyana bandha, feel or see the energy rising up from the root chakra, and lower your chin to meet your chest, corking that energy inside your torso, feeling your body temperature rise slightly. Hold for four seconds, and then release, taking in fresh air.

In the beginning of this chapter, we talked about how yoga could be useful in helping witches know themselves better. Hopefully, after trying out some of the material, you are beginning to get more in touch with parts of yourself that have been ignored in the past. Maybe you felt the energy rise in a way you never have before. Maybe you noticed that your body feels slightly different after trying some of these exercises and practices than it did before. Perhaps you just learned how the breath can help you focus your mind and direct the power. All of these are wonderful takeaways from this chapter. They are all parts of knowing thyself better.

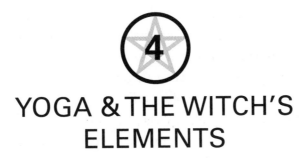

YOGA & THE WITCH'S ELEMENTS

The five classical elements play a part in yoga, just as they do in witchcraft. Patanjali encourages his readers to meditate on the various states of the elements in order to gain mastery over them.[60] In fact, psychic development in yoga stems from mastery over the elements of ether, air, fire, water, and earth. Patanjali ascribes various powers to merely meditating upon the elements. Among those powers are the ability to become smaller than the smallest, creating a sense of wealth, moving through rock, holding one's hand in a fire without getting burned, touching water without getting wet, and standing firm against a hurricane. This is why a great deal of psychic development training starts with a thorough understanding of the elements.

While Patanjali and other yoga sages talk about the elements, they only graze the topic. For a thorough understanding of how a witch can apply the elements to all areas of life, it is essential to turn to Ayurveda. Yoga and Ayurveda are sister practices out

---

60. Stiles, *Yoga Sutras*, 43 (III, 45).

of India that influenced each other greatly.[61] Let's compare the Ayurvedic approach against the Hermetic philosophy of Western occultism.

The Ether

A common practice in both witchcraft and Ayurveda is to address the elements from the most subtle to the most dense. The ether, being the subtlest of the elements, is the source of all the others, and, as such, mastering it is required for success in any higher level spiritual experience. Unfortunately, because it lacks a recognizable shape or image on the physical plane, it is often difficult for our minds to fully grasp this element. Though the Hermetic philosophers address this element, they give very little direction on how to work with it directly. Many witches just rely on the fact that because the other elements have the ether as their root cause, learning to master them will also bring some measure of proficiency with this fundamental element.

Fortunately, this is not the only option available to witches who enhance their practice with yoga or the Ayurvedic understanding of these elements. According to the California College of Ayurveda, ether does have qualities of its own, but, because it is the nature of emptiness, it is often best described by what it is not. Ether is cold, because it lacks the warmth created by fire. It is light, because it lacks the heaviness of water and earth. It is immobile, because it lacks the motion associated with air. Lacking the presence of the other elements, ether is described as the most subtle of the elements.[62]

Sensing the Ether

When I started working with the ether, I had the eerily wonderful realization that this process was similar to how spirits materialize at a séance. We're all familiar with the movie version of this imagery. A group of people gather around a table, holding hands. The lights in the room are dimmed. Maybe it's only lit by candlelight. There may even

---

61. "The Connection Between Yoga and Ayurveda," *Kripalu*, accessed July 15, 2020, https://kripalu.org/resources/connection-between-yoga-and-ayurveda.

62. "The Five Elements: Ether in Ayurveda," *California College of Ayurveda*, accessed July 5, 2020, https://www.ayurvedacollege.com/blog/five-elements-ether-ayurveda/.

be swirls of incense smoke permeating the room. The medium or witch speaks some magick words and calls out to the astral realm for the deceased loved one of one of the other participants. When the ghost materializes in the room, it is transparent. It may even glow a pale grayish-blue color. Objects and even other people can be seen through its body. This is the quintessential example of the etheric energy! During this exercise, imagine that you are the conjured spirit from that movie séance scene.

1. Sit in a comfortable seated position, or, if you can meditate while lying down without falling asleep, lie down flat on a bed or couch.

2. Close your eyes and observe your breath for roughly two minutes. Do nothing else but focus on your breath, watching it rise and fall, slowing it down. Try to make the inhale and exhale equal in length.

3. In your mind's eye, see your physical body as you normally would: solid, dense, and opaque.

4. As you exhale, imagine yourself giving up some of that mass, as if you were breathing it out and growing lighter and colder with each breath. As you inhale, empty your mind. Think of nothing. Simply observe the rise of your stomach and chest as you breathe in.

5. As you are exhaling out your mass, feel your body growing lighter and lighter, colder and colder. Then visualize your body become not only lighter and colder but also less and less opaque until you actually start to become transparent. Without opening your physical eyes, imagine looking down at your body and seeing through it to the ground beneath you.

6. After you have achieved a level of transparency that you are comfortable with and you have experienced the ether for yourself, reverse the process. As you inhale, think about warming yourself up and rematerializing your mass. Do it gradually until you are equally as solid, dense, and opaque as you were at the start of the exercise.

The Element of Air

Air, being finer than fire, water, and earth, is generally addressed next. Like its physical plane manifestation, air's metaphysical aspects are hard to pin down. When addressed in occult texts, air is about motion and exists wherever friction is found. It does not actually have a specific agreed-upon place or order. It stands between the ether and fire in some accounts and between fire and water in others. The truth is that it exists in both places at once.

When talking about the witch's cosmology, Sybil Leek says, "The first step in the process of differentiation occurred in the production of vapor, created by heat, which in time condensed into water. Two elementary forces played their part in these operations: an inward movement and an outward movement."[63] That the vapor in this quote corresponds to the element of air can be seen by the second part of the quote, which talks about the operations. The inward and outward movements are directly related to the motion and friction ascribed to elemental air in other occult texts. This bears out on a mundane level as well. Vapor is another way that we talk about humidity in the atmospheric air.

In the Hermetic philosophy, air is not seen as an element at all. Instead, it is seen as a mediator between the active and passive powers of the fiery and watery principles.[64] Again, we see the essential quality of dynamic friction at work in this philosophy.

The Hermetic understanding to the elements, which has influenced a great deal of modern witchcraft, can be traced back to yoga. Bardon says so in his own discussion of the elements in his book *Initiation into Hermetics*: "In the most ancient Oriental writings the elements are called *tattvas*."[65] On the next page, he goes on to compare his own understanding of the elements against the ancient Eastern philosophy, which, though he doesn't name it, is yoga.[66]

Within Hermeticism air is seen as the principle that establishes a neutral equilibrium between two opposing forces, like fire and water. Air has this quality (and many more) within the Eastern philosophies of yoga and Ayurveda as well. In Ayurvedic

---

63. Leek, *The Complete Art*, 25.

64. Bardon, *Initiation into Hermetics*, 28.

65. Bardon, *Initiation into Hermetics*, 25.

66. Bardon, *Initiation into Hermetics*, 26.

philosophy, air is that "which balances and stabilizes these movements, a force that pulls toward the center (samana)."[67]

Unlike ether, air's effects are easily observed. We can feel the gentle caress of a cool breeze or see a leaf getting carried away on the wind. In historic times, our ancestors were carried across the vast oceans through the power of air. Today, we fly across the same distances through the sky in planes. Our every spoken word is carried on the air. Our breath has the ability to sustain life or excite a lover during a moment of passion. Air is always a force of regulation, something to be witnessed by its effects.

In the Ayurvedic system, air is the primordial, unmanifested form of touch. As such, the skin is the organ associated with this element. The hands, with which we reach out and touch the world, are also connected to this element.[68]

Conscious Breathing (Pranayama)

Both witches and yoga practitioners recognize the inherent power in conscious breathing. Simply by keeping the focus on the breath, you awaken your body's energy. In witchcraft, the breath is often used to direct the energy during a spell—breathing in to collect or raise the energy, breathing out to send the energy toward its intended purpose. In yoga, the focus on conscious breathing is called *pranayama*. During a specific pose or sequence of poses the practice of pranayama aligns the body, mind, and spirit by anchoring the practitioner in the present moment.

Though breathing is an unconscious and involuntary process most of the time, it can be brought under our conscious control for the purposes of magick and psychic development. When you first begin to practice pranayama, it's enough to simply observe the process of your breathing. Lie flat on your back, placing one hand on your belly and the other over your heart.

---

67. "The Five Elements: Air in Ayurveda," *California College of Ayurveda*, accessed July 5, 2020, https://www.ayurvedacollege.com/blog/five-elements-air-ayurveda/.

68. "The Five Elements: Air in Ayurveda."

1. As you inhale, focus on slowing down the breath and breathing deeply into the belly. Feel how your belly begins to expand, like a balloon. Pay special attention to how your body feels as you inhale. What are the initial sensations as you begin taking the breath? How do those sensations change as your belly expands outward? In your mind, ask yourself, "How is this process connected to the element of air?"

2. Pause at the top of the inhalation when your belly is completely filled up. Hold the air for a brief moment, and pay attention to how the sensations have changed. Feel the element of air moving through your body in this moment of pause.

3. As you begin to exhale, imagine trying to touch your belly button to your spine. Don't rush the exhalation. Follow it by focusing on the slow, gradual movement of your hands as the abdominal muscles contract. In your mind, bring up the associations with the element of air again. This time, ask yourself how you are engaging with the element as it leaves your body.

4. Pause at the bottom of the breath, feeling your midsection grow tighter and more compressed. Take a moment and take stock of what it feels like when you are completely empty of breath. How is it different from pausing at the crest of the inhalation? In your mind, ask, "What is it like to let the element of air leave my body?"

After you have become familiar with the mechanical process of how to breathe deeply while lying down, you can try the same exercise sitting up. Over time, you can experiment with sensing the power of your breath in other positions. You can also experiment with different rhythms of breathing and even attach specific thoughts and images to the breath. There really is no end to the variety of ways you can experiment with this exercise once you get the hang of it.

The Element of Fire

Fire is the universal force that transforms one state into another. Its essential qualities are heat and expansion. In addition to those qualities, fire is also heavily connected to the light. Both Hermeticism and Ayurveda[69] admit that "every element of Fire can be transformed into light and vice versa."[70]

Fire contains the essence of the previous two elements within it. Without ether's space to expand into or air's movement to fan its expansive quality, fire would not be able to burn. This is why it is often viewed as the third element in yoga and Ayurvedic philosophies, even though it is said to have been the first among the elements to emerge from the ether in many other theories. Remember that ether lacks recognizable shape and air is always observed by its effects, so they don't generally get recognized before the more dramatic, expansive quality of the fire element coming into being.

Sensing the Fire Element

Kapalabhati is often translated as *skull shining breath* or *skull luster* because the crown chakra lights up the etheric energy around the head. Sometimes this pose is translated as *breath of fire* in English. This is a wonderful exercise to feel the fire within yourself. The belly acts as a bellows, stoking the heat within the torso and allowing it to rise up into the head, which makes the crown appear luminescent upon the astral. This breath is both detoxifying and stimulating.

For this exercise, breathe only through the nose. Focus on the exhale and allow the inhale to happen naturally. Make the exhale longer than the inhale. In yoga classes, teachers will refer to this type of inhalation as a passive inhale. It may take some practice to get used to this type of breathing. In general, people tend to focus on the inhale and allow the exhale to happen naturally. So it may feel a bit unnatural at first, but with a little practice, it will become second nature.

All breathing during this exercise is powered by the navel and solar plexus through rapid stomach pumps. Rapidly pull the belly button tight against the spine as you exhale air through the nose. On the inhale, simply allow the belly to relax.

As you get more familiar with this exercise, your practice sessions can be longer. Some yogis make step 5 in this practice last for a half hour or more before moving on

---

69. "The Five Elements: Fire in Ayurveda," *California College of Ayurveda*, accessed July 5, 2020, https://www.ayurvedacollege.com/blog/five-elements-fire-ayurveda/.

70. Bardon, *Initiation into Hermetics*, 30.

to step 6. However, in the beginning, start with no more than one or two minutes, and build up to more over time if you like.

1. Sit in a comfortable seated position. This can be done in a straight-backed chair or on the floor, but make sure that your spine is fully elongated. Pull the shoulders back and down, away from your ears, and lower your chin toward your chest. It is often enough to simply look down at the ground in front of you. This head tilt does not have to be severe.

2. Close your eyes, and allow your mind to focus on the area between your eyebrows.

3. Touch your index fingers and thumbs together and rest your hands on your knees, palms facing up.

4. Allow yourself to breathe naturally for a few breaths.

5. Now, inhale partway, and as you exhale, begin breathing rapidly. As you do so, focus on compressing the belly button in toward the spine. Allow it to move in with the inhale and release slightly with the exhale. (Think of a dog panting to cool off in the hot summer sun. This is the type of breath you are going for here.)

6. After about a minute or so, take a deep breath in through the nose. Retain the air as long as it is comfortable for you to do so. Then exhale the air out through the nose again.

7. Allow yourself to sit quietly and observe the effects of your practice before you move around.

While this technique has many benefits, one of its main uses is providing mental clarity. It is useful before any spell or ritual that calls upon the mercurial or solar spirits and energies. It's also good to use before casting spells for mental clarity or knowledge of any kind. Again, this is a common pranayama technique, and, as discussed before, pranayama techniques can be dangerous for people with certain medical conditions.

If you have any doubts, please consult a qualified medical professional before trying this technique.

The Element of Water

Water stands as the opposite principle from fire. Whereas fire is hot and expansive, water is cold and constrictive. In its active or positive state, water nourishes and preserves. It's easy enough to see this preserving quality if we look in our kitchens. The coldness of our freezers can preserve food for months when it would have otherwise spoiled. In its passive or negative state, water decomposes, ferments, and disperses.

Bardon tells us that fire and water stand as the two fundamental elements of creation. The fire and ice of the Norse mythologies reflect this occult wisdom. These two elements exist in everything that ever was, is, or will be created. The old-school occultists called fire the electric principle and referred to water as the magnetic principle, and between these two opposing forces, the air element resides as a mediator.[71]

Sensing the Water Element

Yin yoga is perhaps one of the best ways to connect with the water element. It is slow, gentle, and very cooling—very much like the metaphysical qualities of elemental water itself. In this exercise, you will practice a very simple yin yoga pose that has the slow, steady, undulating quality of a peaceful body of water. Imagine standing out on the shore of a lake. As a gentle breeze blows over its calm surface, gentle ripples rise and fall against the edges of the lake where it meets the earth. You will reproduce this gentle motion with your upper body during this exercise.

Your upper body will become like the gentle ripples of the lake lapping at the shore. As you exhale and lower your body, the ripples flow toward the land. As you inhale and straighten your body back up, the ripples ebb back into the lake. It should be gentle and rhythmic.

---

71. Bardon, *Initiation into Hermetics*, 230.

1. Sit with your legs out in front of you. Your knees can be slightly bent or not—whatever is comfortable for your body. Your spine should be straight and your shoulders pulled down away from your ears. This is often called *staff pose*.

2. Gently round the back and roll forward very, very slowly, imagining that your upper body is like the ripples on the surface of the lake. As you exhale, roll your chest and chin down toward your legs. In yin yoga, this pose is called *caterpillar*.

3. On the inhale, gently and slowly reverse the motion, gradually rolling your upper body back up into staff pose. Take the full length of the inhale to come back to the starting position before repeating the rounding motion again on the next exhale.

4. Repeat the process of ebb and flow in line with your breath as you visualize yourself becoming the very water within your imaginary lake.

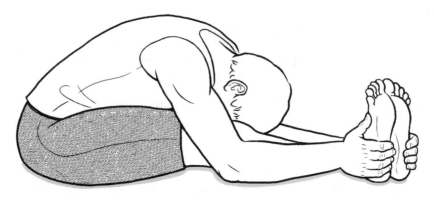

Caterpillar Pose

Allow yourself to continue this exercise as long as it's comfortable for you, lowering gently and slowly on the exhale. Inhaling and returning to the starting position equally as slowly. Be the essence of water. Imagine yourself becoming colder and heavier with each undulation.

The Element of Earth

Like air, earth is not seen as a true element in the Hermetic philosophy. It is an amalgamation of the other elements in various patterns and states of solidity. In order to give concrete form to other elements, they must be slowed down and limited. That is the very essence of the earth element in action. As a result of this limitation, volume, weight, and time come into being. Because it holds the other elements together through reciprocal action, occultists refer to this element as the *tetrapolar magnet*. All the other elements are active within this one, thus it is also referred to as *electromagnetic*.[72] It is the same in the Ayurvedic approach.[73]

Sensing the Earth Element

One of the easiest ways to engage the earth element is to go out into nature, find a tree that calls to you, and sit among its roots with your back pressed flat against its trunk. In my line of witchcraft, we do this all the time. What's interesting is that this same exact practice is said to have been how the Buddha attained enlightenment.

1. Find a good, strong, upright tree. Better that you go out into the woods to do this, but if you are called to a tree on your property, follow your intuition.

2. Talk to it. Touch it. Allow your thoughts to project into it as you do so. If you get any negative feelings at this point, find another tree. If you feel positive and upbeat through this process, take a seat in a simple seated position with your legs crossed in front of you (lotus pose) at the base of the tree.

3. Close your eyes and press your back firmly against the trunk of the tree, making sure that your head is supported so that you may fully relax.

4. Imagine that your tailbone is growing like a taproot and that, as it grows, it travels down toward the heart of the tree. When your taproot connects to the heart of the tree, allow your breathing to sync up with the rhythm of its beating.

---

72. Bardon, *Initiation into Hermetics*, 29.

73. "The Five Elements: Earth in Ayurveda," *California College of Ayurveda*, accessed July 5, 2020, https://www.ayurvedacollege.com/blog/five-elements-earth-ayurveda/.

5. Allow yourself to relax even deeper, thinking of nothing except peace and tranquility. Sit there in quiet contemplation as the tree and you become one.

6. When you lose your focus and become aware of your body again, take a few more gentle breaths with your eyes closed. Thank the tree and the dryad who watches over it, and go about the rest of your day.

This is the beginning of a much deeper form of magick. Once witches master this basic technique, the land around them comes alive and a world of possibilities opens up to them. Pacts with trees, communication with land spirits, interaction with fairies and other elementals—these possibilities and more all open up to witches who learn this basic technique.

The Elements of Occult Anatomy

For us in the West, it is often easier to believe something if we can see results on the physical level first. Western minds are trained to believe that if it can't be proven by science, then it must not be true. This belief actually causes more people to struggle with psychic development than any other belief. After all, mainstream science says magick and psychic powers do not exist, and a foundational occult principle is that energy follows thought. By not believing in the phenomenon until you see the proof that it has already worked, you actually stop the phenomenon from working. Approaching the process psychically, controlling the elements from a physical perspective first, and seeing the positive results of that effort in the body go a long way toward helping Western minds who worship at the altar of science overcome their skepticism.

If you are one of the skeptical scientists, it might be better that you start by understanding the Ayurvedic approach, even though it comes second in this section. There is no psychic exercise for the Ayurvedic approach, since the Ayurvedic section is exclusively focused on the physical aspects of the elements within the body. The Ayurvedic approach is time-tested. It has as much proof regarding the validity of this system as it is possible to get, since it has been successfully in consistent use for over five thousand years.

For witches who do not need proof about the validity of magick and want to jump right to the psychic portion of controlling the elements, the Hermetic approach will help you do exactly that. I put it first in the section because it can work on its own to very good effect, but it can also serve as a boost to your mundane efforts with the physical aspects of the Ayurvedic methods. Getting a handle on the psychic aspects of the elements through the easily visualized system of Western Hermeticism will only help you control your thoughts and direct the energy more effectively.

The Hermetic Approach

Bardon tells us that the earth element rules over the lower body from the feet to the genital organs. Water holds sway over the abdomen region up to the diaphragm or midriff. Air controls the chest with the heart and the lungs, and fire has dominion over the head and all its organs.[74]

Though Bardon focuses a great deal on the mental plane instead of the physical, his analysis of how the elements impact us is worth noting. His understanding helps witches avoid physical problems by balancing these qualities in the mind right as the emotions develop. According to Bardon, when the fire element is out of balance in our minds, traits like jealousy, hate, and anger develop. When we have an imbalance of the air element, self-conceit and wastefulness are present. An overabundance of water leads to feelings of apathy, coldheartedness, and defiance. When the earth element is out of balance, we are easily offended, lazy, irresponsible, and inconsistent.[75] If you notice that you spend a lot of time engaging in any of these emotions, it may be time to reevaluate. After all, you can greatly improve your life simply by changing your perspective on the situations you find yourself in.

Balancing the Elements

While this approach to occult anatomy may seem rather simplistic compared to the Ayurvedic model, I find it useful for visualization purposes during certain exercises, like this one. By connecting large portions of the body to specific elements, it's easier for the mind to visualize the accumulation of elemental energy within the various bodies.

---

74. Bardon, *Initiation into Hermetics*, 127–28.

75. Bardon, *Initiation into Hermetics*, 70–71.

Lie down on the ground or in a bed during this exercise. Take seven deep belly breaths for each element. At the end of the seventh breath, affirm for yourself that you are now filled with the limitless potential of that element for health and well-being. Then begin the next round of seven breaths with the next element, repeating the process until you have completed all five elements.

1. Breathe in the ether. Feel it as a cool weightlessness traveling all over your body. See it as the indigo of a starless night sky.

2. Breathe in the element of fire. Feel it as a dry heat that accumulates in your head, igniting into a halo of pure radiant light by the seventh breath.

3. Breathe in the element of air. Feel it as a gentle warmth that expands the chest like a balloon, making you feel lighter as if you were floating on a cloud.

4. Breathe in the element of water. Feel it as a cold, dense constriction in your abdomen. Let it bring you back down to earth.

5. Breathe in the element of earth. Feel it as a dense heaviness in your lower body. Feel yourself sink into the ground beneath you.

Take a few moments and allow the energy to go where it needs to in order to heal the body. When you're ready, open your eyes.

The Yoga & Ayurvedic Approaches

While each element is responsible for different structures within the physical body, just as they are in the Western version of occult anatomy, the Ayurvedic system is not quite as linear in its approach. Instead of declaring that the earth rules over the lower body, the water influences the belly, and so on, the Ayurvedic approach looks at the structures of the body holistically. All regions of the body are composed of various combinations of all five elements.

According to the California College of Ayurveda website, "The five elements represent the most important foundational concept in Ayurveda."[76] Like Bardon's Her-

---

76. "The Five Elements in Ayurvedic Medicine," *California College of Ayurveda*, July 4, 2020, https://www.ayurvedacollege.com/blog/five-elements-ayurvedic-medicine/.

metic version, each element corresponds with different parts of the body and mind. Unlike Bardon's placement, the Ayurvedic approach ascribes the elements to structures or functions within the body, not regional areas.

Ether exists within the hollows of the physical body. The empty intestines, the blood vessels, the bladder, and the lungs are all filled with ether. When the ether is counteracted or corrupted, it results in an increase in space and a decrease in structure, which results in the destruction of bodily tissues.[77]

Air within the body is deeply connected to motion and the life force in general.[78] It controls the circulation of blood and the rhythm of the breath, among other things. It is the force that impels all movement. There are actually five forms that the air takes in ancient Vedic texts, and all are related to motion. It can move inward, outward, up, down, or it can be the force that balances and stabilizes the other movements by moving to the center.[79] "Air may move too fast, too slow, or become obstructed and blocked. Each occurrence produces different effects depending on the location of the air that is disturbed."[80] Should you desire to balance the air element within you, start with the basics. Maintain a steady routine that promotes good health. If you have too much air, balance it with a heavier meal. Air is always pacified by engaging the other elements.[81]

In Ayurvedic medicine, fire evolved out of ether and air, just as we saw in Sybil Leek's account of the witches cosmology earlier in this chapter. Ether gives fire the space to exist and air propels it into motion, fanning the flames, so to speak. Like air, fire has five distinct expressions within the body. Fire regulates the metabolism and helps us digest food, but it also ignites the mind, helps us see, energizes the body, and radiates warmth from the body outward.[82] When there is an excess of fire, the skin breaks out in rashes and inflammation is more likely to occur. When there is a lack of fire in the body, the metabolism slows down, the skin loses its luster, and the mind

77. "The Five Elements: Ether in Ayurveda."

78. "The Five Elements: Air in Ayurveda."

79. Ibid.

80. Ibid.

81. Ibid.

82. "The Five Elements: Fire in Ayurveda."

becomes sluggish.[83] The easiest way to tend the fire within the body starts with monitoring the metabolism. You can increase the fires of digestion by consuming hot, spicy, sour, or salty foods. Conversely, decreasing the fire element in reference to metabolism can be done by consuming heavy and cold foods.[84]

Water contains aspects of the other three elements, which is why it comes fourth in this system. Ether provides it with a container in which to exist. Air gives water its ability to flow. As the heat of fire cooled and condensed, water came into being. When maintaining one's health, water is the antidote to symptoms caused by opposite qualities. According to the California College of Ayurveda, "It is important to take in the qualities of water when you are feeling too warm, ungrounded, emaciated, dehydrated, rough, lacking in self-esteem, obstructed and immobile, irritable with a sharp tongue, transparent and vulnerable, or if your heart has become too hard."[85]

Earth contains all the other elements in this system, just as it does in the Hermetic philosophy. It represents all that is solid and material within the universe. Even the physical components of the other elements are earth. The pattern of the wind, fire's flickering flame, the physical water we drink—these qualities came to pass because of the earth element. The earth element is also responsible for the solidity and form of the body. The easiest way to control the earth element within the body is through the diet. Earth energy is found in large amounts in grains, nuts, legumes, and meats. It is found in moderate amounts in dairy, fruits, vegetables, and spices. Therefore, if you want to increase the earth element within the body, eat foods with large quantities of this energy. If you want to decrease the influence of the earth element, eat foods with moderate amounts.[86]

By balancing the elements within your body in a physical way, you will eventually see how your efforts pay off psychically. As we saw when discussing the water element within the body, this method of elemental control influences the emotional and

---

83. Ibid.

84. Ibid.

85. "The Five Elements: Water in Ayurveda," *California College of Ayurveda*, July 5, 2020, https://www.ayurvedacollege.com/blog/five-elements-water-ayurveda/.

86. "The Five Elements: Earth in Ayurveda," *California College of Ayurveda*, July 5, 2020, https://www.ayurvedacollege.com/blog/five-elements-earth-ayurveda/.

mental planes as well as the physical. Consuming water helped regulate the heat of the body, but it also soothed sharp fires of an irritable tongue and worked its magick on the hardened heart. Over time and with enough success regulating your body and mind through the simple suggestions for balancing the elements given in this section, even the most skeptical observer will find it hard to deny the validity of this occult science.

Putting Them Both Together

The belief that our thoughts and emotions will eventually impact our health is central to both the Western Hermetic approach and the Eastern Yogic and Ayurvedic approaches of occult anatomy. However, this process works in reverse, too. The gift of physical health is just the beginning for witches who practice controlling the elements as part of their psychic development.

By balancing the elements within the body, witches can gain control over their minds as well. There's a very simple reason for this. Consciousness and ether both share the same subtle qualities, because ether is consciousness. Neither one can be observed directly. They also lack substance or form. In being nowhere specific, they are both omnipresent. The other four elements, being various combinations of the ether, are merely different manifestations of consciousness. This understanding of the elements aligns with the Vedic wisdom surrounding the concept of *maya*, which says that the world is an illusion within the mind of a Supreme Deity.[87] This approach also aligns with the Australian Aboriginal concept of the Dreamtime.

In order to master the elements for psychic development, it is important to understand the basics of how they interact. Their relationships are governed by natural laws, and these laws hold sway equally on the physical, emotional, and mental planes. The elements can either support, destroy, or cooperate with each other. Dr. Swami Shankardev Saraswati, a Western medical doctor with yoga and Ayurvedic credentials,

---

87. "The Meaning of Maya: The Illusion of the World," *American Institute of Vedic Studies*, July 20, 2020, https://www.vedanet.com/the-meaning-of-maya-the-illusion-of-the-world/.

wrote an excellent introductory article explaining the interactions of the elements for *Yoga Journal* back in 2007:[88]

1. Fire and water are said to "destroy" each other if they come in contact. On the physical plane, this happens when we quench a fire. Though the flames go out, the water evaporates just as quickly. This is one of the reasons why Bardon sets his simplified occult anatomy up with air in between the water and the fire.

2. Some elements are actually supportive of each other. Air and fire increase each other's influence. Think of the concept of fanning the flames. Water and earth are said to "hug" each other. Think of mud. Both water and earth are coexisting without either trying to overcome the other.

3. Other elemental combinations are referred to as *cooperative*. They neither support nor destroy each other. For example, air and water function well together without creating problems, but, given the chance, they will separate. Fire and earth are the same way.

Learning to apply those laws to the elements within their own physical bodies and minds helps witches bring order out of chaos physically, emotionally, and mentally. Once witches strike an internal elemental balance, they can begin working their wills on the world around them.

Achieving a Mental Equilibrium

Energy follows thought. So far in this chapter, you have accumulated the elements within your astral body and balanced them within your physical body. Now, it's time to balance the elements within the mind. After all, it doesn't do any good repairing the physical damage if your mental state will only repeat the process.

To master the elements on the mental plane, you need to begin a process of self-analysis. Go through every personality trait you can identify.

---

88. Swami Shankardev Saraswati, "Purifying the Five Elements of Our Being," *Yoga Journal*, July 20, 2020, https://www.yogajournal.com/teach/purifying-the-five-elements-of-our-being.

1. During the first week, jot those personality traits down in a list. This list should be made up of both good and bad qualities. Don't think about it. Don't judge that list. Just keep adding qualities to the list. It's okay to repeat qualities or to say the same thing in different ways. Just keep adding to the list.

2. During the second week, clean up that list. Rephrase things. Polish it up. Eliminate all the repetitive qualities. Divide the list between the good and bad qualities, so that when you are done you have two lists—one of your strengths and one of your weaknesses.

3. Ascribe elemental associations to each quality on both lists. For example, if you are quick to anger or determined, that would be a fire quality. Thoughtlessness and joy are qualities associated with the air. Shyness and compassion are water in nature, and the earth rules over things like laziness and integrity. On some level, the elemental associations are subjective, and you may need some time coming up with the elemental associations for some of the mental qualities on your list. However, if you are honest with yourself and you understand the nature of each element, you will be fine. Use the descriptions of the elements from earlier in this chapter to assist in your deliberations.

4. Once you have completed your two lists and ascribed elemental associations to every mental quality, take four more pieces of paper. Label each of the pages after the elements—air, fire, water, and earth. Also draw a line down the center of each page, creating two equal columns. In the left-hand column, write the word *Positive*. In the right-hand column, write the word *Negative*. Then begin dividing your list of qualities up between each of the four pages, putting the personality trait under the proper element in its assigned column.

5. Ideally, your lists should be exactly equal and filled with positive qualities. No one element should dominate your consciousness for either good or ill. However, that's rarely how it happens for most people. Most of us tend to favor one element over the others.

6. If you find yourself with an imbalance between your lists, begin by transmuting the qualities in the column marked *Negative*. Follow the Ayurvedic guidelines

for how the elements interact. For example, it is easier to transmute a negative fire quality into a positive air quality. The two work well together. If you can't find a suitable air quality, the second best option would be to look for a quality ruled by the earth element. In very rare cases, it might be appropriate to convert that fire quality into a watery one. However, you will have to do a great deal of work in the transmutation process; remember that these elements fight each other whenever they are closely aligned. After you have transmuted all the negative qualities you can, it is appropriate to begin swapping positive traits between elements if a balance still needs to be achieved.

This whole process should take you about a month if you're diligent in your efforts.

Magick & the Elements

Many of these truths regarding the elements and their ordering, as they are described in yoga's cosmology, are mirrored in the typical placement of the elements within the Circle-Cross format of the witch's Circle Cast. The version of the witch's Circle that I am referring to here ascribes the elements to the quarters, placing air in the east, fire in the south, water in the west, and earth in the north. There are certainly other effective ways of ordering the witch's Circle. If another version calls to you, feel free to use it instead, but I prefer the Circle-Cross setup because of one particular wisdom that it reveals.

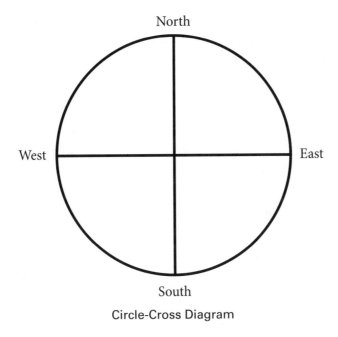

Circle-Cross Diagram

When witches use this format to cast the Circle clockwise or deosil, as some witches say, they are mimicking the explosive process of creation on a microcosmic level. The Circle goes from subtle to the most condensed, gaining greater solidity as the witch moves from the east through the south and back to the east again. The energy of this Circle is projective, and it mirrors the moment of the big bang, which expanded outward from the Void into existence. This is one reason that witches in my tradition only cast our Circles deosil when we wish to cleanse or banish something from a space. Tarostar, one of the elders within my branch of witchcraft, talks about this concept in his book *The Sacred Pentagraph*. He says, "Deosil is a positive gesture and positivity banishes that which is already there."[89]

In Hermetic philosophy, this energy is referred to as *electric* or the *electric fluid*. The electric current is also talked about as being *positive* in nature. Like earthly electricity, the metaphysical electric current has fire as its source, and like the fire element itself, it is expansive in nature. The expansive quality of the fire element explains why many

---

89. Tarostar, *The Sacred Pentagraph: A Craft Work in Five Volumes: Books I, II & III* (New Orleans: Left Hand Press, 2015), 170.

witches describe seeing the Circle as a bubble. The electric nature of a deosil Circle also accounts for the drastic difference in temperature between the witch's Circle and the world outside of it. Bardon tells us that "fire with its expansion into all directions has warmth as its specific attribute and is therefore spherical."[90]

Whereas the electric current has the fire element as its source, the opposite current originates with water. It is referred to as *magnetic* or the *magnetic fluid* in Hermetic philosophy. Because of its attractive quality, the magnetic current is talked about as being *negative* in nature. The Circle-Cross model of the witch's Circle Cast accounts for this energy as well. When witches cast their Circles counterclockwise or widdershins, they are creating a magnetic current. Tarostar also says, "Negativity attracts to itself"[91] so "…to create a Magic Circle for any form of occult work which is to call and attract a specific Force, a widdershins motion should be started."[92]

By casting the Circle widdershins, moving from the north and working through the west back to the north, witches create a magnetic or negative current that attracts the etheric forces to their ritual or spell so that the accumulated energy may be programmed according to their intention. Where the electric or positive current is characterized through expansion or banishing, the negative or magnetic current has constriction or attraction as its primary quality. The widdershins Circle functions more like a vortex, funneling or attracting the surrounding energy into its center. While the image used to envision a deosil Circle is often the bubble, I tend to imagine a Circle cast widdershins more like a whirlpool. This is just another example of the law of balance at work within the witch's magickal practice.

Positive & Negative Thoughts

As any wise witch will tell you, magick doesn't just happen within the Circle's boundaries. It's part and parcel of every aspect of a witch's life. The action of casting the Circle actually mirrors the way we think.

---

90. Bardon, *Initiation into Hermetics*, 101.

91. Tarostar, *The Sacred Pentagraph*, 168.

92. Tarostar, *The Sacred Pentagraph*, 170.

Just as the Circle may be cast in a positive or negative current, the mind can be filled with positive or negative thoughts. In addition to all its other benefits, the Circle-Cross format also explains the reason why people who keep their minds focused on the positive side of things seem to sail through life more easily. This approach to witchcraft also explains why people who keep their thoughts focused on the negative, always worrying about the worst-case scenario or feeling discouraged or angry all the time, just seem to have it so much worse than other people do.

The positive current banishes what was already there, while the negative current attracts that which is like it. This works on all planes of existence—the physical, the energetic, the mental, and so on. That means that when you are faced with adversity and you choose to keep your thoughts positive, you are actually working an act of magick, cleansing your mental landscape and banishing your burdens. However, when you allow your mind to dwell on your fears and worries, you only attract more of what you're focusing on. You actually draw that fear or worry into your life just by dwelling on it. You are effectively cursing yourself.

To see the truth of this theory, try this simple exercise. Next time you find yourself in an uncomfortable situation, stop. Take three deep belly breaths. Clear your mind of all doubt and worry. Simply focus on your breath, like you did in the conscious breathing exercise from earlier in this chapter. When your mind is clear, think of a desirable outcome to the situation. Then think of things that make you happy—time spent with loved ones, a good meal, the best gift you've ever been given, cuddling your pet. Anything will do. All that's important is that your thoughts make you truly happy. When you have achieved a genuine moment of happiness, open your eyes. Repeat the process as often as you need to until you get through the uncomfortable situation.

Do this often enough and you'll notice that "bad" things happen to you less and less often. You'll also start to notice that "good" things begin to happen more and more frequently. Things just seem to start going your way. People are nicer to you.

If that doesn't convince you and you're a glutton for punishment, try the reverse process. I dare you. When an uncomfortable situation presents itself, imagine the worst. Dwell on your anger and fear. Get as upset about it as you can. Maybe even co-opt friends into your misery and talk as much trash as you can with them. Then take notice of the results.

Let me be clear. I do not recommend this second method. However, if you absolutely need to see both sides of the situation to convince yourself not to allow your thoughts to dwell in the negative current in the future, then the little bit of pain this will cause you in the present may be worth it.

———————

A thorough understanding of the five elements is essential to a witch's psychic and magickal success. While modern Western occult philosophies, like Hermeticism or Theosophy, give witches a good entry into exploring the role of the elements in their practices, the Western approach often leaves some important questions unanswered. Yoga and its sister practice of Ayurveda can be extremely useful in filling the information gaps.

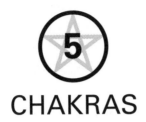

CHAKRAS

As valuable as yoga was in deepening the witch's understanding of the five classical elements, there is still so much more wisdom to be gained from studying the parallel paths of witchcraft and yoga together. After the elements, a study of the chakras will bear the most fruit. Understanding these energy centers within the subtle bodies can help witches get a better handle on how to use their bodies to raise energy more effectively as they work magick and develop their psychic powers.

Today, it seems like everyone is talking about the chakras. On social media, they are a hashtag. They are a keyword for internet searches. Businesses use them as part of their brands. Sometimes it seems like you can't turn a corner without running into them. There are entire books written about the chakras. I've seen chakra-themed merchandise, like chakra-based clothing and singing bowls.

Western fascination with the chakras isn't a new phenomenon. It didn't just start when Facebook or Instagram became popular. People were fascinated by the chakras back when the Theosophists introduced them to the Western world in the nineteenth century.[93] During the later part of the twentieth century, society embraced the chakras

---

93. Leland, "The Rainbow Body: How the Western Chakra System Came to Be," 25–29.

on a mass level, and the interest has been steadily growing since the 1970s. In Initiatory Wicca, or British Traditional Witchcraft as it is sometimes called, the ritual practice referred to as *The Fivefold Kiss* lines up remarkably with several of the well-known chakras and some of the minor or lesser-known chakras as well. By kissing various points on a partner's physical body, a witch is opening up the partner's chakras in the subtle body with the sacred breath. The feet, the knees, the genitals, the chest, and the lips all align with chakras in various Vedic descriptions.

Even people who don't get into any other form of occult or magickal practice simply adore the chakras. I remember when I started my yoga teacher training, there was this one devout Christian woman who just loved yoga, but she couldn't tolerate all "that heathen nonsense" that studying yoga beyond the gym made her learn. She had a problem with kundalini. She detested the mythology behind the practice. The constant reference to Hindu texts made her feel like she was betraying her God. However, she did not have a problem with the chakras. In fact, she loved them. When I asked her how she squared that with her faith in the Christian God, she said, "God doesn't make mistakes, and if He gave me chakras, there must be a reason." Ultimately, she dropped out of the program because she saw it as conflicting too much with her worldview, but her willingness to embrace the chakras when she railed against everything else was fascinating to me. I'm not sure what it is about them, but the chakras just seem to bridge spiritual party lines in a way that almost nothing else does.

The Chakras in Yoga

The ancient Hindu writings are confusing when it comes to describing the chakras. Unfortunately, the internet and modern social media have only compounded that confusion. For a witch who wants to work with the chakras in a structured energetic practice, getting access to valid information can often be quite difficult. Even experts, like Mark Stephens, the author of *Teaching Yoga*, admit to struggling with the confusion surrounding this topic. He says, "As with everything in the world of yoga, with chakras there are numerous contrasting and even conflicting views about what they are, how they work, their number, location, and even whether location is a relevant concept."[94]

The seven chakra model, which most people are familiar with, has its origins in an eleventh century tantric text. The *Sat-Cakra-Nirupana* was written by a Bengali yogi named Purnananda. It was one of the first texts to discuss the topic of the chakras, describing them as emanations of divine consciousness.[95] Within its pages, Purnananda teaches the reader to raise the kundalini energy in order to attain realization.

"We know this book was highly esteemed through the centuries because it was the subject of numerous commentaries."[96] The most famous Western commentary on this book came from Arthur Avalon (Sir John Woodroffe) in his 1919 book *The Serpent Power*, which reprinted a full English translation of Purnananda's original text. It is still one of the standard resources on the topic for Westerner yogis to this day.

Because of its historical value and the sheer volume of commentary available on it, referring back to Purnananda's *Sat-Cakra-Nirupana* can give us a foothold toward clarifying some of the confusion surrounding the chakras. Purnananda directly addresses the chakras, how many of them there are, and their location.

One of the more fascinating aspects of the *Sat-Cakra-Nirupana* is that even though it is credited as a possible origin of our modern understanding of these energy centers,[97] it only describes six chakras—the root, sacral, navel, heart, throat, and third eye.[98] Purnananda did not talk about the crown chakra directly. However, he alludes to it. Avalon references another text in backing up Purnananda's wisdom. He says, "See the opening verse of Paduka-panchaka: 'I adore the twelve-petalled Lotus that is the crown of the Nadi along the channel (Randhra) within which the Kundali passes.'"[99] He mentions it

---

94. Stephens, *Teaching Yoga*, 55.

95. Ibid.

96. Purnananda Swami, "Sat-Chakra-Nirupana," accessed July 23, 2020, http://www.bahaistudies.net /asma/7chakras.pdf.

97. Stephens, *Teaching Yoga*, 55.

98. Arthur Avalon (Sir John Woodroffe), *The Serpent Power* (India: Ganesh & Co. LTD., 1950), 317–64.

99. Avalon, *The Serpent Power*, 324.

by name in the next paragraph (*Sahasrara*) while explaining the theory being discussed in the *Paduka-panchaka*.[100]

In the preliminary verse of Purnananda's text, he says, "Now, I speak of the first sprouting shoot (of the Yoga plant) of complete realization of the Brahman, which is to be achieved, according to the tantras, by means of the six Chakras and so forth in their proper order."[101] In his notes on the commentary of this first verse, Avalon says, "According to Shankara, by 'other things' are meant the Sahasrara, etc."[102] *Sahasrara* is the sanskrit word for the crown chakra, and Shankara is one of the more renowned commentators on the *Sat-Cakra-Nirupana*. As Avalon's translation shows, Purnananda did account for the crown chakra, though he didn't articulate its value within the system. That means that, on some level, the seven chakra system dates back as far as the eleventh century.

Avalon's commentary on Purnananda's text can also be used to address the conflicting information around whether location is relevant to the chakras. In verse 1, Avalon explores different theories before he goes on to give Purnananda's actual wisdom. Avalon goes into great detail about the nadis in relation to the spinal column.[103] In analyzing Purnananda's first verse, Avalon locates the nadis in specific locations within the body. The initial investigation starts out by exploring the relationship between the nadis and the spinal column, called *Meru* in Sanskrit.[104] Avalon tells us that some theories place the Ida Nadi to the left of the Meru and the Pingala to the right.[105] He talks about how some theories describe them as being "shaped like bows"[106] and how the two nadis, which come from the left and right scrotum, meet with the Middle Pillar. According to this version of occult anatomy, Avalon tells us that the nadis then make a plaited knot when they reach the eyebrows before proceeding down to the nostrils.[107]

---

100. Ibid.

101. Avalon, *The Serpent Power*, 317.

102. Avalon, *The Serpent Power*, 319.

103. Avalon, *The Serpent Power*, 320–64.

104. Avalon, *The Serpent Power*, 321.

105. Ibid.

106. Ibid.

107. Avalon, *The Serpent Power*, 322.

He talks about the nadi that comes from the left scrotum, bows around the heart, and passes onto the right nostril, and how the nadi that originates from the right scrotum bows similarly while passing onto the left nostril.[108] After exploring other theories to back up his point, Avalon turns his attention to Purnananda's theory. He says, "Our Author speaks (in the following verse) of the Lotuses inside the Meru."[109]

In verses 2 and 4, Purnananda goes on to describe the actual location of various chakras within the physical body. He says that the *Sushumna* is "subtle as a spider's thread, and pierces all the Lotuses, which are placed within the backbone."[110] In verse 4, Purnananda tells us that the root chakra or muladhara is "attached to the mouth of the Sushumna, and is placed below the genitals and above the anus. It has four petals of crimson hue. Its head (mouth) hangs downwards."[111] Not only do the chakras seem to have a distinct location within the body, they also seem to face specific directions— at least for Purnananda and his translator, Avalon.

Location of the Chakras

Though Avalon's translation and commentary on Purnananda's text does much of the heavy lifting in resolving many of the discrepancies surrounding the chakras, the debate is far from over. The conflicting information that Stephens mentions within the world of yoga is equally as compelling as Avalon's interpretation of the *Sat-Cakra-Nirupana*. As witches, though, we have a resource for resolving the discrepancies that does not often get considered in the more traditional yoga discussions: personal psychic experience.

While yogis traditionally discourage conscious psychic development, many witches treat psychic training as foundational to their spiritual paths. It is the acceptance of the personal gnosis gained through those personal psychic experiences that makes all the difference in how the witch approaches the conflicting information on topics like the chakras.

In addition to consciously trying to develop psychic powers, witches take great pains to study the phenomenon that they experience during their training sessions.

---

108. Ibid.

109. Avalon, *The Serpent Power*, 323.

110. Avalon, *The Serpent Power*, 327.

111. Avalon, *The Serpent Power*, 331.

This unabashed acceptance of the psychic life allows witches to understand the etheric double in a way that most yogis never consider, and that firsthand experience can shine the light of wisdom through the confusion about the number and location of the chakras. Regardless of where the chakras correspond to on the physical anatomy, they do actually reside within the etheric body, and discussing the etheric body can be confusing even between adept occultists who otherwise agree. For example, both Blavatsky and Besant had different opinions regarding this principle of humanity, despite the fact that they were both Theosophists. Blavatsky placed the etheric body between the vital body and the lower manas.[112] Besant thought it belonged between the physical body and the vital body.[113]

One of the reasons that so many experts disagree on number and location of the chakras is because the etheric body does not always align perfectly with the physical body. Many people tend to think of this body as a duplicate of the physical body. Even the Theosophists had a tendency to talk about it that way. Both Blavatsky and Besant referred to it as an astral or etheric double on several occasions, and while it can be an exact replica of the physical body at times, it is not always so. In its natural state, the etheric body is a bit like an amorphous, ambient cloud that permeates and surrounds the human body—maybe something like what clairvoyants typically describe when looking at someone's aura or how ghosts are said to be able to coalesce before the viewer's eyes.

The fact that the etheric body can, but does not always, take the same shape as the physical body accounts for many of the discrepancies in the various texts regarding the chakras. By accepting the malleability of this body, accounts that used to appear contradictory can be reconciled. Witches who approach the etheric body and the chakras from this fluid perspective gain access to a greater storehouse of occult wisdom and techniques to work with the chakras and advance their psychic development much more quickly.

When the etheric body does take the exact same shape as the physical body, the chakras do line up in the commonly accepted place. The root chakra (muladhara) exists at the center of the pelvic floor. The sacral chakra (svadhishthana) is about two

---

112. Blavatsky, *The Key to Theosophy*, 53–55.

113. Besant, *The Seven Principles of Man*, 10–15.

fingers' width above the root chakra. The navel chakra or solar plexus (manipura) resides about two fingers' width above the belly button. The heart chakra (anahata) occupies the center of the chest. The throat chakra (vishuddha) is positioned in the pit of the throat around the thyroid. The third eye (ajna) resides around the center of the forehead, and the crown chakra (sahasrara) is located at the top of the head.

Working with the Chakras

Have you ever heard someone talk about "activating" their chakras? If so, did you wonder what they meant by that? I know I did.

For the longest time, I had heard about this practice, but nobody could explain what was actually happening on a mechanical level behind that catchy little phrase. It never actually made sense to me. That is, it never made sense to me until I began comparing my yoga and witchcraft training.

When using the standard seven chakra system, there are two ways to approach the chakras. The system can be approached by starting at the root and working your way up to the crown, or it can be approached from the top down. When approached from the root up, this is referred to as activating the chakras. It's just a fancy way of talking about opening them up to receive energy in order to activate the chakra's influence on your life.

However, merely activating or opening a chakra is not enough. Once the chakras are open, they also need to be charged with universal energy. This practice actually mirrors the process of manifestation talked about by the Theosophists in their theory regarding the Seven Principles of Man. Just like matter becomes more and more dense as it descends through the seven planes of existence, knowledge and wisdom become more and more conscious as they descend down through the chakra system from crown to root.

Many Valid Chakra Systems

Despite what our Western occult history teaches us, the truth is that there isn't just one version of the chakra system in traditional yoga. There are many. Like the various branches of witchcraft, each yoga tradition has its own preferred system and understanding for dealing with the chakras. What's even more fun is that all of them can be right at the same time.

As much as I love the Theosophists and I appreciate their assistance in bringing many Eastern traditions to the attention of the Western mind, I have to admit that many of them, like C. W. Leadbeater, did not stick to traditional interpretations on the chakras when they wrote about them. This is not a condemnation of their efforts, just a statement of fact. That fact should not be used to discredit their work, however, since different theories exist harmoniously within the various traditions of yoga.

Even in the most traditional systems of yoga, the sages and scholars admit that the chakras are focal points for meditation. The material provided by Western occult writers, like the Theosophists, did help people engage the chakras in meditation, and the collective experiences of those people did bear out consistent similarities over time. For that reason, there's no reason to consider their efforts invalid, just because they deviate slightly from some of the more traditional sources. Remember, the chakras exist within the etheric body, and the etheric body is mutable. It can coalesce around and change in response to human thought. Because the etheric body is fluid and the chakras belong to the etheric body, their position within that body is also fluid. The chakras do not exist in a fixed position. They move and flow with the etheric body itself. There are more or fewer chakras depending on the thoughts and intentions of the person meditating on them. Therefore, it really doesn't matter which version of the chakra system you work with, whether you see five chakras, seven, or hundreds. If you understand the foundational concepts of the particular system you're using and you adhere to that system faithfully, you will get the results promised by that system.

Admittedly though, there are a few chakras that appear in every system, regardless of tradition. They are the sacral chakra, which governs sex and creativity; the heart chakra, which governs love and compassion; and the crown, which governs understanding and our path to enlightenment. Even in systems that don't acknowledge the crown chakra directly, like Purnananda's, there is still a hat tip to this chakra, and those systems tend to associate these areas of influence with the third eye. You might notice that these three chakras are heavily connected with the three most common places where people talk about getting psychic impression: the gut feeling that cops often talk about, a mother's intuition that comes from compassion for her child (often associated with a heaviness or tightening in the chest), and the precognitive under-standing that generally gets associated with the head.

The Chakras & the Elements

In most Western accounts of the chakras, each chakra has an elemental association. The root chakra is associated with earth. The sacral chakra is associated with water. The solar plexus is associated with fire, and the heart chakra is associated with air. However, just like all the other associations, these correspondences are completely arbitrary.

When most Westerners practice chakra visualizations, they are taught to repeat specific mantras to concentrate their minds on a desired thought. A mantra is a word or phrase that gets repeated either verbally or silently to yourself, which focuses the mind during meditation. Mantras are very similar to the witch's charms and spells. Many people teach mantras in connection with the specific chakras. They'll say that the word *lam* is the mantra that is associated with the root and focuses the mind on that chakra. The sacral chakra mantra is *vam*. *Ram* is the mantra for the solar plexus, and *yam* for the heart. However, these associations are also entirely arbitrary.

The words being used as mantras are actually associated with the elements, not the specific chakras themselves. The word *lam* is associated with the element of earth. *Vam* is associated with water. *Ram* is associated with fire and *yam* with air. They have only become associated with specific chakras because the elemental associations have been added into our Western understanding of this system. They are not necessarily con-nected in this way, and it is possible to work with the chakras without the elemental associations. In fact, it is often preferable to work with the chakras independent of their standard elemental associations. Working with the chakras actually becomes a much more robust energetic practice when you disassociate the mantras and their cor-responding elements from the specific chakra.

Think about this for a moment. When healing through the elements in witchcraft, witches know that too much of any one elemental energy in a person's energetic field can cause untold problems. This applies to the elements within each individual chakra as well. Take, for example, the association of the earth element with the root chakra. One of the primary associations with the root chakra is evacuation of the bowels. What happens if too much earth energy is applied to that area? How "blocked up" does the situation become? Consider the case with the element of fire as well. Too much fire energy in a person's energetic field can cause inflammation. As witches, we know that in order to heal inflammation, we must balance that fire energy with its opposite. Can you imagine what always having fire in the solar plexus (the center associated with digestion) would do to a body? Consider the effects of this abundance of fire energy on a nonphysical level. The solar plexus is the energy center associated with personal power in the seven chakra system. How many super egos have been fanned by the flames of this association? Bikram Choudhury, the infamous yoga teacher who, according to many different sources, including the most recent documentary on Netflix, terrorized his students to no end, immediately comes to mind. What would happen if someone who was struggling with keeping their ego in check were to bring the compassionate power of water or the grounding influence of earth energy into the solar plexus instead?

The Root Chakra (Muladhara)

When most people in the West think of the root chakra, their minds immediately drift to the topic of sex. They think this is the energy center that governs their sexual passions, desires, and lust. It is not, but the confusion is understandable, because its area of influence does overlap slightly. The root chakra is all about our foundations—survival, security, and our basic needs. It's the basic needs piece that makes people associate sex with this chakra, but that's not, strictly speaking, a good association. The root chakra is more concerned with issues of reproduction and survival of the organism and the species than any one individual's particular sexual appetites. That facet of our lives comes into play with the next chakra in the system.

When the root chakra is in balance, the person is strong and expresses self-confidence and the rest of the chakras in the system stand a better chance of operating effectively. This should probably be the first place you look when problems arise, because, even if the issue exists in another chakra, it probably has its foundation in something to do with the root chakra.

When the root chakra is out of balance or blocked, the individual can become unstable—expressing neediness, insecurity, and suffering. Ultimately, these conditions trace their own origin back to low self-esteem. When a root chakra is extremely out of balance, the person in question may even engage in destructive behaviors. If you are dealing with insecurity, fear, or a lack mentality, this chakra may hold the key to overcoming those struggles.

Root Chakra Symbols

There are some common symbols that will help you focus your mind on this chakra during meditation. They are the following:

- The color red.

- This lotus flower has four petals. Each of the petals on the flower corresponds to one of the four aims of human life (Dharma, Artha, Kama, and Moksha).

- The Hindu god Shiva in his guise as Pashupati, the Lord of the Animals.

- The elephant.

The Sacral Chakra (Svadhishthana)

The sacral chakra is the center of self and creativity. This is where the sexuality that most people identify with a healthy adult lifestyle actually comes into play. It is the place where desire and the procreative drive merge into sexuality. This chakra is also the seat of much that qualifies as *subconscious* in modern psychology.

When paired with the physical anatomy, it is easy to see the power of this chakra. It is about movement. In his book *Yoga of the Subtle Body*, Tias Little says, "Within the pelvis, [the sacral position] plays a pivotal role as centerpiece at the back of the pelvis, permitting movement through the sacroiliac (SI) joints. As part of the spine, it forms the base of the spine and acts like a rudder, helping to stabilize and steer the entire vertebral column."[114]

The fact that the sacral chakra is positioned between the root chakra and the solar plexus tells us something else. It operates as a sort of crossroads, mediating between the base animalistic awareness of the root chakra and the personal empowerment associated with the solar plexus. This liminal connection also sheds light on why some

---

114. Tias Little, *Yoga of the Subtle Body: A Guide to the Physical and Energetic Anatomy of Yoga* (Boulder, CO: Shambhala Publications, 2016), 75.

systems of yoga only recognize three chakras, with this one serving as the base in those systems. It combines elements of the root and solar plexus.

Sacral Chakra Symbols

There are some common symbols that will help you focus your mind on this chakra during meditation. They are the following:

- The color orange.

- This lotus flower has six petals. The petals on this lotus are traditionally seen as obstacles to be overcome in order to purify the chakra. They have been listed as anger, hatred, jealousy, cruelty, desire, and pride.

- There are two Hindu deities associated with this chakra. They are Brahma (a creator god) and Saraswati (the Hindu goddess of wisdom, art, music, and learning).

- The crocodile.

The Solar Plexus Chakra (Manipura)

The Sanskrit word *manipura* has been translated as *lustrous gem, palace of jewels,* and *city of jewels* because it is said to shine bright like the sun to clairvoyant people. Supposedly, this chakra is the most radiant and glowing of all the energy centers. In line with that translation, the solar plexus shares in the resplendent qualities that many witches associated with the solar energies. It is the center of willpower, personal empowerment, self-esteem, and vitality.

This chakra is all about transmuting energy from the lower chakras in order to build power. The root chakra provides the raw material. The sacral chakra churns or moves that material around. The solar plexus transmutes the lower forms of energy into power, which is why it is often translated as *power center* in many texts.

Again, looking at the physical anatomy to understand the metaphysical can be useful here. Tias Little says, "Through the evolution of biological structure, all creatures whether the triceratops or the tree frog, an alligator or an armadillo, a shark or an inchworm, never expose their bellies. For animals to expose any part of their front is to make the organism vulnerable to the risk of attack."[115]

Solar Plexus Symbols

There are some common symbols that will help you focus your mind on this chakra during meditation. They are the following:

- The color yellow.

- This lotus flower has ten petals. The petals on this lotus are traditionally seen as distractions that, if indulged, can disempower the individual. They are sadness, foolishness, delusion, fear, disgust, shame, treachery, jealousy, ambition, and ignorance.

- The Hindu god associated with this chakra is Rudra (the howler). He howls with passion and ecstasy, guiding us toward our higher calling.

- The ram, which hints at similarities between this chakra's associations and the traditional correspondences of the sun sign Aries in astrology.

The Heart Chakra (Anahata)

Whereas the previous chakra was all about personal empowerment, this chakra is relational. The heart is the center of connection. It deals with empathy, compassion, partnership, our connection to others, and, ultimately, love.

The various English translations of the Sanskrit word *anahata* reveals one of its deepest secrets and the source of this chakra's immeasurable impact on our lives. The word *anahata* has been translated as *unstruck*, *unbeaten*, and *unhurt*—referencing the fact that the core of this chakra remains untouched by the trauma we go through in life. It vibrates at such a high frequency of love that none of the struggle and strife of this world can touch it, which means that no matter how bad things might appear to be in the present moment, there is always a way to transcend the situation.

---

115. Little, *Yoga of the Subtle Body*, 103–4.

Heart Chakra Symbols

There are some common symbols that will help you focus your mind on this chakra during meditation. They are the following:

- The color green. Sometimes green with a pink center.

- This lotus flower has twelve petals. The petals on this lotus flower represent twelve potential mental disturbances that, left unchecked, can impair our consciousness and make us less loving. These disturbances are lust, fraud, indecision, repentance, hope, anxiety, longing, impartiality, arrogance, incompetence, discrimination, and defiance. By meditating on these disturbances (called *vrittis* in Sanskrit), the heart chakra is balanced and a person's full capacity to love is restored. This restoration applies equally to self and others.

- The Hindu deity connected to this chakra is another aspect of Shiva referred to as *Ishana*. Some accounts say both Shiva and Shakti dwell within this chakra together.

- The deer or antelope.

The Throat Chakra (Vishuddha)

Many experts will tell you that this chakra is about communication, and so it is. However, it is also so much more than that. This is actually the chakra of expression. Expression is more than just verbal communication. It is the act of bringing an internal experience or way of knowing out into the world around you. Expression can happen as a solitary process. Nobody necessarily needs to witness your truth in order for you to be able to express it. Communication, on the other hand, only happens when someone else is there to receive it.

This chakra's Sanskrit name has been translated as *especially pure, to purify*, and *completely pure*, which hints at the fact that this chakra is the source of Udana or upward-moving breath. Udana directs prana from the lower chakras up into the higher. As it moves, Udana purifies the body of toxic substances. This is yet one of the reasons why yoga teachers always remind their students to focus on the breath. It is purifying. However, that purification isn't just detoxing the body. It's doing the same thing to the mind by cleansing the subconscious of all the things we've "swallowed down," "stomached," or in some other way failed to fully express.

Have you ever heard someone call another person *true blue*? That phrase hits at a very core concept surrounding this chakra, and it also explains why this chakra has been associated with the color blue. *True blue*, as a phrase, refers to a person who is unwavering and fully committed to a particular cause. In order to be able to express oneself authentically, a person must first be true to self.

Throat Chakra Symbols

There are some common symbols that will help you focus your mind on this chakra during meditation. They are the following:

- The color blue.

- This lotus flower has sixteen petals. The meaning ascribed to each of the petals for this chakra's lotus have been greatly debated by various traditions, but all the meanings seem to revolve around a similar theme: expression of ability over time. Within various yoga philosophies, the petals of this chakra lotus are associated with the *kalas*—powers and abilities expressed by Lord Krishna in Hindu mythology.

- The Hindu deity connected to this chakra is Panchavaktra Shiva. His skin is blue and he has five heads, each one representing a different sense.

- The white elephant.

The Third Eye Chakra (Ajna)

The Sanskrit word *ajna* has been translated as *obey, authority,* or *command*, which is only appropriate as this chakra governs the functionality of all the other chakras. The third eye provides insight and transcendent wisdom. The ideal is to lead one's life in alignment with the wisdom gained by engaging this chakra. By working more with this chakra, people are put on the paths that are most appropriate for their own unique purposes.

When this chakra is balanced, people become more insightful and their intuition becomes more powerful. When this chakra is blocked, people become closed-minded and distrusting. They will also focus too much on logic.

Most people associate the third eye chakra with the region of the face between the two eyebrows. This is because novice meditators are taught to focus on that spot, which is called a *kshetram* in the yoga world, in order to activate their third eye. As the novice becomes more adept at meditating on this chakra, though, the kshetram becomes less of a focal point and the attention shifts further back into the skull to the point where the spinal cord and the skull connect. The physical anchor for the third eye is actually the pineal gland, which exists right at the same level as the eyebrows. There is no danger in using the kshetram, and it will not negatively affect your meditations on this chakra if you choose to keep your focus on the eyebrows instead of the back of the skull.

Third Eye Chakra Symbols

There are some common symbols that will help you focus your mind on this chakra during meditation. They are the following:

- The color indigo.

- This lotus flower only has two petals. They represent the Self and God.

- There are no Hindu deities associated with this chakra.

- This chakra also lacks an animal association.

The Crown Chakra (Sahasrara)

The crown is the last of the seven primary chakras in this system. This is the point where the Self gives way to what Western occultism calls *The All* and what some witches might call the deity that exists above the God and Goddess. The Sanskrit name for this chakra, *sahasrara*, means *thousand* or *infinite* for this reason. This is the point of connection within a person's energetic body where the finite taps into the infinite.

Crown Chakra Symbols

There are some common symbols that will help you focus your mind on this chakra during meditation. They are the following:

- Some traditions see this chakra as violet. Others see it as white. Personally, I prefer the white visualization, because it connects with so many of the meditations in witchcraft. For example, when we pull down the pillar of light in the Middle Pillar exercise during the Lesser Banishing Ritual of the Pentagram (LBRP), we are tapping into this chakra.

- This lotus flower has a thousand petals, which represent the full blossoming of consciousness.

- There are no Hindu deities associated with this chakra.

- This chakra also lacks an animal association.

Though the chakras originally stem from ancient Hindu texts, they have worked their way into witchcraft through a variety of sources, and there is good reason for this. The chakras help witches gain better control over their etheric bodies, which are extremely fluid and often difficult to imagine without clearly defined imagery to focus the thoughts. The chakras and their various correspondences give witches that clearly defined imagery.

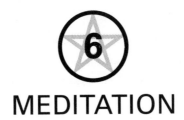

MEDITATION

"I can't meditate."

I've heard this particular mantra countless times before—both as a yoga teacher and as a witch, and never once has it actually been true. The truth is, everyone can meditate. Everyone.

Meditation does not have to happen while you are sitting on the floor with your legs crossed in front of you and your hands neatly folded in your lap. That's only one version of meditation. Meditation can be done lying down on your bed, walking around outside in nature, while you're cooking dinner, or while you're waiting for an appointment at the doctor's office. Meditation can be done anytime.

Let me show you.

A Simple Meditation

Right now, in this present moment, we're going to meditate together. After you're done reading through these instructions, put the book down and think. It doesn't matter what position you're in. It doesn't matter whether you're sitting, standing, or lying down. It also doesn't matter if your eyes are opened or closed. Just consider all the times you get bored in any given day. Run through a catalogue of your past week, and conjure up incidents where you were bored. Some examples might be times when you were waiting for a phone call or when you were standing in line at the grocery store. Just remember those events. That's it. You don't have to do anything else. Just remember. When you feel satisfied that you have found enough, open your eyes.

Guess what. You just meditated!

It really is that simple. This does not have to be some grueling process. We all meditate all the time. It's the idea that this is one more thing we have to make time for or that it is something to be practiced that turns so many people off. Our lives are busy and stressful enough. We don't need to give ourselves one more thing to struggle over.

The good news here is that, when it comes to meditation, you don't have to struggle and you don't have to find extra time to do it. All those moments you just remembered are already ideal points in your schedule to add in a simple meditation, like the one you just did. Rather than be bored, antsy, frustrated, or something else, why not concentrate on something specific for a few moments and give yourself a well-deserved break from the daily grind? As you saw in this meditation, it doesn't matter if your eyes are opened or closed. Meditation can be done either way. It's really just concentration. Sometimes it's concentration on a series of thoughts, like what you did here. Sometimes it's concentration on a single thought, and sometimes it's concentration on removing all thoughts from your mind. At its most simple, meditation is just concentration.

––––––––

Meditation: The Heart of Witchcraft

I have been training people to meditate for most of my adult life. The connection between a yoga teacher and a meditation coach is already firmly established in the minds of most people in the West. I don't need to spend much time dwelling on that. However, the connection between witchcraft and meditation is less firmly established in the minds of witches new to the Craft.

Most people who start out on the witch's magickal path get drawn in by the spells and the idea that they will be empowered to change their lives for the better. Few of these people actually associate this empowering skill with meditation. It seems like they think about meditation as an Eastern practice, something only Buddhist monks or yogis do. It can often come as quite a surprise to these people when they find out that meditation is at the very heart of the witch's magick. They often have a difficult time wrapping their minds around the idea that nothing in witchcraft can be done without it. Psychic development, spells, rituals—they all require a basic level of skill with meditation.

Meditation is at the very heart of witchcraft. Like yoga with its eight limbs, some branches of witchcraft also have an eightfold path. This path has been called *The Eight Ways to Center* by some witches, while others have simply called it *The Eightfold Path* or *The Eightfold Way*. According to Lady Sable Aradia's book *The Witch's Eight Paths of Power*, "In his *Book of Shadows*, Gerald Gardner writes about the witch's Eightfold Way as a means of developing one's magickal abilities."[116] The eight ways to raise power discussed in this model are the following:

1. Meditation or concentration

2. Trance or astral projection

3. Rites, chants, spells, runes, charms, etc.

4. Intoxicants (incense, wine, etc.)

5. Dancing and kindred practices

6. Blood and breath control

---

116. Lady Sable Aradia, *The Witch's Eight Paths of Power* (Massachusetts: Weiser Books, 2014), back cover.

7. The scourge

8. The Great Rite

Meditation is listed as the first of these eight ways because it is involved in all the others. Without the power of concentration, trance simply does not happen. Failing to achieve the ecstatic trance state also eliminates the possibility for astral projection. Without concentration on a specific intention, lighting candles is just burning wax, nothing more. Without forming a mental image and concentrating on its fulfillment, rites, chants, and so on are just moving around a circle performing predetermined physical actions. I could go on, but I think the point is clear. Meditation is essential to witchcraft.

———————

If you are like most new witches and you struggle with the idea of meditating, let me tell you two brief stories about two witches I have trained who also struggled with this concept. The first witch professed that she absolutely could not meditate. When I kept pushing the issue, she got belligerent with me in defense of her stance that meditation was beyond her. She even went so far as to poke fun at the idea of meditating. When I didn't back down to her aggressive tactics, she then started to justify to me why she was right and I was wrong.

At first, she tried to give me medical reasons why she couldn't meditate. Then she changed course and tried to tell me that her mind just moved "way too fast." She tried to explain that she simply had too many important responsibilities that prevented her from navel-gazing.

When I didn't buy what she was selling, she went on the attack, trying to make the issue about me. She said things like, "Not all of us can afford to spend our days teaching yoga. Some of us have to work for a living," and worse, but when I didn't back down, she finally just admitted the truth. Meditation was boring, and she hated the idea of it.

One day, while we were talking on the phone, she brought up the fact that she took a bath each night. When I asked her why she made time for that, she said that it helped her unwind. Knowing that this was my way into the discussion on meditation again, I began asking her some pointed questions about her nightly ritual.

"Do you listen to music, or is it silent?"

She told me that it was usually silent because the rest of her day was crazy busy and everyone and their mother wanted to talk to her. This was her time to turn off the noise and just relax. It was her chance to take care of herself.

Check.

"Do you sometimes replay the events of a particularly stressful day in your mind before you let them go?"

She confirmed that she did.

Check.

"After you let them go, do you find that you experience a deep sigh of relief and your muscles just seem to relax in the warm water?"

Again, she confirmed that I was describing her situation.

"Aha!" I shouted into the phone.

"What?!"

"You're meditating!"

There was silence on the other end of the phone. I genuinely thought she had hung up on me, because the silence lasted so long. When she finally did speak, she was overjoyed. It was like watching a child learn to read or ride a bike for the first time. For the next few weeks, it was all she could talk about. She compared everything to meditating in her bath.

The second witch tried the same tactic with me. Truth be told, it was almost as if he were reading from the same exact script, although his performance was more convincing that the first witch's. He had depression and OCD, and I had to understand that sometimes that meant he just couldn't force himself to do something. He ran a successful business, and sometimes that meant he had to drop everything when his clients called. Like the first witch, his mind moved "way too fast." He couldn't ever hold just one thought at a time. He was constantly being bombarded by all the things he had to do in a day. Important things were already getting shuffled to the back burner. He didn't have time to "just sit there." His mind and his life simply didn't work that way, and I had to accept that, or so he thought.

Just like I did with the first student, I let this witch say what he wanted to say. I just listened to the excuses and empathized with his plight. Then one day, while we were talking on the phone, he told me a story about what life would be like if his business were successful enough that he could do everything he ever wanted to do. When he started his story off with, "I just want to take my morning coffee out on my porch and relax without having to worry about deadlines," I knew I had found the trigger that would give him his own moment of inspiration.

As the conversation went on, he fought me, but that was to be expected. He had invested a lot of energy into the idea that he couldn't meditate. He wasn't just going to give it up because I said so. He needed to be the one to convince himself that he could meditate.

That said, when I have an agenda, I'm like a dog with a bone. I may not know how I'm going to achieve my goal, but, once I slip into that mindset, I have absolutely no doubt that I will eventually succeed. In my heart, I truly felt this was my moment to help him over this particular hurdle. To be perfectly honest, he had annoyed me with his protestations that he simply could not meditate for a few months by this point, so I may have taken a bit more delight in pressing the issue than was, strictly speaking, necessary.

"Roll with me here for a moment," I said. "Close your eyes."

He confirmed that he did.

"Now, imagine yourself on your porch on that glorious morning when you have finally achieved the success in your business that you just talked about."

I waited for him to confirm that he had conjured up the image in his mind.

"See yourself sitting at that round glass top wicker table in one of your wicker porch chairs with the comfy cushions."

Uh oh! He was definitely in for it now. I had been to his house several times, because we are in the same tradition. I knew his house like I knew my own. I could paint the scene picture-perfect, and he was already going along with my imagery. I could hear his breathing pattern change through the phone. It was slowing down. It was clear that he was actually seeing the imagery in his mind.

"Now, grab your coffee cup."

"Mmmmmmm …" he sighed as I continued to paint the picture.

"As you take a sip of your coffee, I want you to think of something. Anything. It doesn't matter what you choose. Take a moment and let an idea come to your mind. Then tell it to me."

He told me, and I immediately came up with a thought that was opposite the one he chose. Then I told him to hold both thoughts in his mind, and I repeated the quote by Aristotle about the mark of an educated mind is the ability to hold a thought without accepting or denying it.

As part of my instructions to guide him through his meditation, I told him how just entertaining both thoughts at one time and refusing to choose between them qualified as meditation. I told him that he didn't even have to close his eyes to do it. He could just sit there on the porch with his morning coffee, sipping away as he contemplated an idea, and that would absolutely qualify as meditation. Then, just to turn the screw a little tighter, I said, "By the way, as you have sat here and listened to me, you have been meditating."

There was silence on the other end of the phone. He later told me that he just sat there stunned with his eyes wide open, like a deer caught in a car's headlights.

After he regained his composure and starting laughing about his own surprise, we broke down the experience. He expressed how delighted he was to know that there were different ways to meditate, that it could happen doing something he loved, like drinking his morning coffee on the porch. He had always loved that Aristotle quote, which I knew because he had told it to me on several occasions in the past. He had also loved Einstein's stories about being able to hold two opposing thoughts, and I knew this as well. So I figured, why not use them? I play to win, folks!

Since their breakthroughs, neither of those two witches has struggled with meditation again. In fact, they have both gone on to try more traditional styles of meditation with great success. The male witch whom I described has even started doing yoga as a result of his *aha* moment.

———————

Again, meditation is the foundation of witchcraft. If you're not able to meditate, then you also aren't able to do witchcraft. If you're one of the people who struggle with meditation, don't let that bother you, because there is good news.

"The good news?" you ask?

Meditation doesn't have to be what you think it is. It does not necessarily have to be emptying your mind. Like the two witches described in this chapter found out, meditation can be done around any activity you already enjoy doing—a bath, your morning coffee, anything. You don't have to lie down or sit on the floor with your legs crossed. Meditation doesn't need you to carve out separate or special time just for it. It can be as simple as replaying the events of your day and releasing the tension associated with those experiences as you exhale, like the first witch did with her bath. It can also be more like the two thoughts meditation I led the second witch through. You can just contemplate two opposing thoughts at one time until you lose your concentration on that topic.

In addition to being good for witchcraft because it strengthens the powers of concentration, meditation also brings some amazing health benefits. It reduces stress, which, according to the Centers for Disease Control and Prevention, is linked to at least six of the leading causes of death and accounts for 75 percent of all doctor visits in the United States.[117] Meditation uplifts the heart and elevates the mood. In truth, it is actually the best medicine for negative emotions. If you're feeling down, meditate. If you're nervous, meditate. If you're angry, meditate. Depressed? Meditate. You get the idea. Though most people associate meditation with a calm, peaceful feeling, it also has the quality of providing an instant burst of energy when needed. Meditation just seems to do it all.

---

117. S. P. Simmons and J. C. Simmons, *Measuring Emotional Intelligence* (New York: Summit Publishing Group, 1997).

A Meditation for Well-Being

We've seen how meditation connects with both yoga and witchcraft. We've talked about it in reference to the chakras and used the power of concentration to turn breathing into a magickal experience. We've even seen some simple meditations in action.

Now, let's try a more structured and targeted meditation practice. This meditation is designed to clear the chakras of difficult emotions, beliefs, or behaviors that block your energy and negatively impact your ability to be successful and happy in the present moment. During this meditation, you will pinpoint the chakra where your particular pain or discomfort resides. It does not matter whether that pain is affecting you spiritually, mentally, emotionally, or physically. Once you find the pain, you are going to hold it there with a specific hand gesture so that you can concentrate your thoughts on it without losing your focus or intention. These hand gestures are called *mudras* in yoga.

The specific mudra that we will be working with in this meditation is called the *Rudra mudra*, and it has so many wonderful benefits. Among its many benefits is the fact that it eases tension and promotes mental clarity as it empowers the individual to achieve a specific intention. To perform this mudra, simply touch the tips of the ring and index fingers to your thumb while extending the middle and pinky fingers comfortably. In general, this can be done with one hand or both hands.

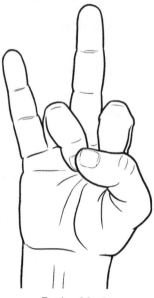

Rudra Mudra

1. Create a mantra that you can repeat out loud to yourself. Make sure to have a specific intention in mind as you create the mantra. For the sake of simplicity, let's say your intention is to get control of your anger. To create this mantra, you must do two things.

   • Negate the negative state, which, in this case, is anger. Something like, "Anger has no power over me."

   • Replace the negative state with an opposite positive condition. Maybe you'll choose something like, "Anger dissolves away easily and effortlessly, leaving me feeling peaceful and content."

   So, for our example, the whole mantra would be, "Anger has no power over me. It dissolves away easily and effortlessly, leaving me feeling peaceful and content." Take some time on this step. You'll need to repeat the process for your specific circumstance.

2. Now, close your eyes and scan your body with your mind. Look for the place where your anger is residing. Anger generally is described as a tension or a heat. Some people talk about it as if their chest has tightened up. Others will tell you that they feel their blood boil or they feel "hot under the collar." The sensation and the location of the anger may be different for you than it is for other people, so pay attention to your own body's natural response to where this emotion is located.

3. Place your hand on that chakra center. It may not be the first place where some sources tell you that anger (or whatever emotion you're working with) is "supposed" to reside. Many people will tell you that rage resides in the root chakra and love resides in the heart, but remember the etheric body where the chakras reside is more fluid and malleable than the physical body. You may be holding your anger someplace else. For example, in step 2, anger could have been in the root, the solar plexus, the heart, or the throat chakra. It just depends on how your body is processing it at that moment.

4. For this specific exercise, perform the Rudra mudra with both hands over the chosen chakra.

5. Now, with your hands in place, see a white light a few feet above your head. Let that light descend through your chakras (first through the crown, then to the third eye, the throat, the heart, the solar plexus, the navel, and, finally, the root). As the light passes through each chakra, say your chosen mantra out loud to yourself and take two deep belly breaths before moving on to the next chakra. When that light gets to the spot where you are holding your hands over the pain, see that light burn that pain away, like a laser beam. See that chakra begin to glow brighter and ignite into flame, burning away the pain. As the pain catches fire within your mind's eye, see the light transmute it into the positive emotion(s) you chose in step 1. In this case, that would be peace and contentment. If you need to, you can put images to the emotions. Whatever you do, do not move on from this chakra until the light has burned up the negative feeling and you feel the shift in your consciousness, no matter how

slight that shift might be. Once you do feel the shift happen, though, carry on to following the light through the remaining chakras.

6. Repeat as often as needed.

By giving your mind visualizations to focus on and your hands something to do, we have taken away much of the sting of meditation. Most of the time when people struggle to meditate, the struggle stems from boredom or a wandering mind. The boredom and the tendency to wander can both be fixed with specific instructions meant to lead your mind through a narrative or story.

————

Whether you're adept at meditation or you're absolutely convinced that you can't meditate, the exercises given in this chapter will help you make progress in your psychic development. Again, absolutely everything in witchcraft begins with meditation, but meditation doesn't have to be lazy navel-gazing. It can merely be a mental shift in how you approach activities you already love doing—going for a walk, taking a bath, or drinking a cup of coffee.

VISUALIZATION, IMAGINING
& ASTRAL TRAVEL

There is a good reason why the subtle body gets so much attention in both witchcraft and yoga. Not only is knowledge of the subtle body useful when working energetically with the physical body, it's also the key to psychic development. What most people call psychic powers are actually inner senses connected to or channeled through the astral or etheric body.

There are two classes of psychic powers: the abilities originating from within the astral body itself and the ones channeled through it from the higher planes. For example, clairvoyance is often called astral sight because it is the ability to look through the eyes of the astral body and see the astral realm; however, telepathy operates above the astral on the mental plane. It is merely directed through the astral matrix to the physical body of the telepathic witch.

Just as there are five physical senses, there are also five corresponding psychic or inner senses. Just like clairvoyance is seeing through the eyes of the astral body, clairaudience is hearing through its ears. Clairsentience is feeling through the astral body. These three subtle senses are well known to most people. The last two remaining senses are less well known. Clairalience is the ability to smell through the astral body.

This is often described by people who smell a mysterious fragrance on the air, like when someone inexplicably smells a deceased loved one's perfume after a funeral. Clairgustance is the ability to taste with the astral body. Though this ability is less often talked about than the other four, we have a subconscious memory of it. Phrases like *that leaves a bad taste in my mouth* harken back to this ability. People who randomly taste foods or flavors without having consumed anything on the physical plane are experiencing effects from this psychic sense. This sometimes happens to mediums during séances.

The protean nature of this body, which was discussed in this book's chapter on the chakras, comes into play here as well. Just as the astral body can manifest and reabsorb chakras, it can do the same with things like eyes, ears, a mouth, hair, and so on. Being mutable, the astral body conforms itself to thought. This is actually how the witch's glamour works. A witch concentrates on a specific effect, and the astral body of that witch responds to the witch's thoughts and will to produce the desired change. Without the witch's attention on the astral body, it resolves itself back into its natural state, as was already discussed. In order to gain astral sight or any of the other inner senses, the witch must first concentrate on that sense and willfully engage the astral body to see through its eyes. Witches who are able to see visible phenomenon in the physical world around them have merely gained the ability to align the astral eyes with the eyes of the physical body. The same holds true with the other senses.

Some psychic abilities, like telepathy, empathy, intuition, precognition, and so on are even more subtle than the inner senses of the astral body. Their further degree of subtlety could be one explanation for why it is often so hard to explain the insight gained through them. The fact that these abilities aren't connected to any sensory organ within the physical body or the astral matrix might also account for why their information presents as impressions or intuitions. Not being connected to a particular sense, sensory descriptions fail to do their wisdom justice.

Most books that address the topic of psychic powers start witches off with exercises for developing clairvoyance, telepathy, or some other psychic sense. If you've struggled with the standard psychic development exercises, there is another approach that may prove more effective for you. Learning to understand the astral body and how it functions in relation to the other bodies (physical, mental, etc.) can only help witches gain control of these abilities faster and more effectively.

The Foundational Skill: Imagining

Many of the more advanced psychic powers have their roots in one simple foundational skill: visualization. If you struggle with visualization, you must work on developing this skill more fully now. Your future psychic success depends upon it.

Before we get to the visualization techniques though, let's clear up a common misconception about the act of visualizing. The name is unfortunate, because it's misleading. Despite the name, mental visualization is not purely a visual experience.

Mental visualization is actually more like imagination, which is why I prefer that title. In order to "visualize," you must engage all five senses on a psychic level. It's a lot like daydreaming. Just like daydreaming, visualization is easy. You just relax and let go as you drift between waking consciousness and slumber. During a daydream, you engage all five senses, which combine to create a realistic experience that, for a time, can rival the waking world consciousness. It's the same with a mental visualization. In order to be convincing, you must engage all five senses and really experience the thing you are imagining. In witchcraft, this complete belief in the imagined experience is often discussed as *intention*.

Imagining

Here is an exercise to help you experience your subtle inner senses. Take your time with this. It is a foundational skill and well worth mastering. Try it with a few different objects. If you don't like lemons, replace the lemon with a fruit you do like. Just make sure to engage all five senses in your exploration of the different objects.

Go ahead and close your eyes. Start by simply focusing on your breath. Allow yourself to be peaceful with your eyes closed for roughly two minutes. Just relax and allow your thoughts to focus on your breathing. After about two minutes, imagine yourself standing in your kitchen. See yourself pick up a lemon. Notice its bright yellow color. Now, roll the lemon around in your hands. Feel its bumpy skin against your palms. Feel its shape within your hands. Turn it around a few times. Look at it from different angles. Now, grab a small cutting board and a knife, and cut the lemon. See the zest gush up as the knife penetrates the lemon's skin. Smell the lemon's fragrance. Cut through the lemon and hear the sound of the knife slicing through the lemon. Feel the knife hit the cutting board. Does it make a sound? Now, take the lemon and sink your teeth into the lemon's flesh. Taste it. Enjoy it.

If you were able to experience all those sensations, then congratulations! You have just engaged all of your astral senses and gotten one step closer to developing your psychic powers. If not, don't beat yourself up. It takes time to reawaken the astral senses, because we have been trained to ignore them for so long. Repeat this exercise every day for a week or two. Stay consistent in your practice, and, eventually, you'll experience the full scope of sensory experiences on the astral plane as you do on the physical plane. It just takes some time and effort.

The Fear of Astral Projection

Once a witch begins to gain some proficiency with the imaginative will and intention, the next step in psychic development is to actively engage the subtle senses in their natural environment. In order to do this, a witch must succeed at getting out of the physical body and into the astral body. This is why astral projection is often referred to as an *out-of-body experience.*

Unfortunately, there are a few fears that can often present problems or stumbling blocks to many beginning projectors. These fears often shut down the experience before it happens. Remember, the astral body responds to thought. If you're afraid of projecting or leaving your body, you will not be able to consciously do so easily. Many of these fears can be alleviated by a simple explanation of how the mechanics of astral projection actually work.

Being Locked Out

Some people fear that if they succeed at getting out of their physical bodies during an astral projection experience, they may not be able to get back in. While this fear is certainly understandable, it develops from a misunderstanding of the astral projection process. The alternative name for astral projections, *out-of-body experiences*, also contributes to the perpetuation of this fear in many people.

You do not actually leave your physical body during an astral projection … at least, not all of you. This fear can be alleviated by a simple modern analogy. Think about astral projection more like the process of creating a PDF on your computer.

While you're working with a file on your computer, it is stored as a different type of file on your hard drive—a file containing written words, a spreadsheet, or some other master document. When you are ready to share it with someone else and you want them to see it exactly as you saw it, you convert that file into a PDF. Then you send it over the internet, through your email inbox to theirs. Just because the PDF has traveled through the internet doesn't mean that it ever left your computer's hard drive. Rather, a replica was made of that PDF, and that was sent off to venture out and interact with the world.

Let's say that one or more of your contacts decides to make a change to that document. They would revert the PDF to its original format, make the necessary changes to the document, and then convert it back into a PDF once again, which they would email back to you. When that PDF comes back, you download it from your email to your computer's hard drive. After looking it over and assimilating the new information, you decide whether to accept that information or discard it into your computer's trash bin. If you accept it, the file can be used to modify and update the original master document. The next time you create a PDF of that master document, it will have the previously made changes as a part of it when it ventures out.

Though this is a simplified example, it is accurate and accessible enough for most people to overcome the fear of astral projection on this account. Your physical body is never left empty, like a shell. It always has some of your energy left behind in it, like the master document, keeping it fully alive and functioning while your consciousness becomes aware of another plane of existence.

Being Replaced

The fear of someone else stealing or taking over your physical body is similar to the fear of not being able to get back into the physical body after an astral projection. This fear is actually rather prevalent. In fact, it's so common that Anne Rice wrote a book about it titled *The Tale of the Body Thief*, which was published in 1992.

The PDF analogy just discussed also speaks to this fear, though. Because the physical body is never left as an empty shell, and because some part of your energy is always present within it, even while you astral project, there is no need to fear having your body stolen.

Death of the Physical Body

Another common fear is that the physical body will die as a result of astral projection. The persistent nature of this fear is mostly because modern occult writers fail to make a distinction between the vital body and the other energetic bodies. By acknowledging the difference between the vital and astral bodies, witches simply do not have to fear that they are leaving the physical body unattended to wither in place as they journey out upon the astral. The vital body never leaves the physical form while it is alive.

For witches who do yoga, this fear is easily alleviated. By engaging the vital body through pranayama techniques, witches gain awareness of the vital body's subtle energy, distinct from other forms of meditation and concentration. By feeling their own vitality increase and surge through their bodies during the asana portion of a yoga practice and feeling energized for hours afterward, witches who practice yoga also learn to feel the effects of the vital body's influence on the physical body.

The Silver Cord

The famed silver cord always comes up in discussions when people talk about physical bodily death as a result of astral projection. This topic gets a lot of attention online, but outside of that arena, I have never heard a reputable account of someone actually seeing their own silver cord during an astral projection. I do not personally believe in the silver cord, but there are several possibilities for what this silver cord could actually be.

1. The silver cord might be a metaphor for the pull that the physical body has over the astral body. When a witch has projected out of the physical body but remains in close proximity to it, the physical body does seem to exert some magnetic pull over the astral double. Some people have described it a bit like the snap of a rubber band or a string being tugged.

2. It might be a blind meant to scare the uninitiated from attempting to get access to the astral realms. The ability to project really is that useful in helping a witch develop psychic powers!

3. The most likely possibility is that the silver cord is an example of Christianity creeping into the occult. The King James version of the Bible says this about the silver cord: "(6) Or ever the silver cord be loosed, or the golden bowl be broken, or the pitcher be broken at the fountain, or the wheel broken at the cistern. (7) Then shall the dust return to the earth as it was: and the spirit shall return unto God who gave it."[118] This is the only original source material I can find where the silver cord is mentioned directly.

If you have had your own personal experience with the silver cord, you must honor that gnosis and operate intuitively in whatever way brings you comfort and peace of mind concerning your own health and safety. Unfortunately, I have nothing to give you on this account. In all the times I have safely projected, I have never once seen my own version of this fabled tether. More to the point, when I have spoken with other witches whom I respect about this topic (and I have talked with many), they have also expressed bafflement over the concept of the silver cord.

Vulnerability during a Projection
A witch recently asked me if he needed to put up any protections in order to astral project. The short answer to his question is no. The longer answer is that basic common sense rules apply. If you're going to put yourself in a meditative state, it's always wise to lock the doors and turn off your phone or other electronic devices in order to prevent unnecessary disturbances. You don't want to be jarred out of your peaceful meditative experience. These mundane world precautions are generally enough for the witch just starting out with astral projection.

That said, peace of mind is essential. If you are worried for the safety of your physical body, your emotional well-being, or your mental health, this fear will present some obstacle to you being successful with your efforts to project. If either mundane or

---

118. Eccles. 12:6–7 (King James).

magickal protective precautions help you feel more comfortable during the projection experience, you should use them.

There are countless books on charms, amulets, talismans, and other protections that witches can make to secure their safety during projections. Some of them can be worn on the witch's body. Others can be used to protect a specific space. Both are useful in making you feel more comfortable during your astral projection experience. It might be worth exploring your options before moving on to step 3, but since they are not essential to the process, I won't spend much time on them here.

What I will say is the charms, amulets, talismans, and so on within books are meant for exactly this purpose. They work their magick upon the astral. The himmelsbrief of the Pennsylvania Pow Wows and the Sator Square of Roman antiquity are two really wonderful examples. Though they are both hung on the walls of your home here on the physical plane, their protective magick works upon the astral. Approaching a house with one of these protections is a very different experience when journeying through the astral realms than it is on the physical plane.

Fear of Harm to the Physical Body

Fear of physical bodily harm is probably the one fear mentioned so far that is the most grounded in reality, but it is not as dire as it sounds. There are certainly accounts of physical sensations occurring because of astral projection. However, just because you experience something stabbing you or you get shot with a gun on the astral does not mean that you are going to come back to your physical body to a hemorrhaging wound. The way it works is a bit more subtle and complicated than that.

In order to navigate this fear, it helps to return to the Theosophical discussion regarding the Seven Principles of Man, discussed in chapter 2 of this book. The spiritual, mental, and emotional bodies are all more subtle than the astral, which, in turn, is more subtle than the vital or the physical bodies. When the astral body projects out of the physical body, it takes the subtler energy bodies—the emotional, mental, and spiritual—with it. Basically, what that means is that your awareness of the emotional, mental, and spiritual aspects of your consciousness turns away from the physical and is focused instead upon the astral journey.

Being that the emotional and mental bodies are more subtle then the astral body, they are "contained within" it during a projection. That means that the emotional and mental states of a person's consciousness can be affected by the events experienced during an astral projection. Upon reintegrating the astral body back into the physical body, those emotional and mental experiences also get reintegrated, and they can influence a witch's daily life for good or ill, just as if they had happened in normal waking consciousness.

This is actually the foundational concept behind many branches of Eastern medicine, like Ayurveda. Most physical ailments start in the emotional body. If the negative emotions persist long enough, they tend to manifest as physical symptoms or diseases. If they are addressed and resolved while they are still emotional, however, the physical body remains largely unaffected. So, yes, it's possible for harm to come to the physical body through an astral projection experience. However, astral projection is no more dangerous than interacting with other people online or in the physical world. The important piece here is that if something bad does happen on the astral plane, you have time to fix it before it manifests as a physical symptom or condition.

Protection & Safety

If you are ever scared or uncomfortable during one of the dreaming exercises, it is important to remind yourself that you are dreaming and that nothing there will hurt you. The only difference between the dream you are currently having and every other dream in the past is that you are conscious of the fact that you are dreaming in this one. Remind yourself that though nightmares have been unpleasant in the past, they have never caused physical harm to you, and neither will this experience. Then take a moment and recollect your thoughts.

Developing the ability to maintain the critical faculty while asleep is part of the lucid dreaming experience, and most of the time that will be enough to put you back in control. Though if you want a little extra guarantee, you can always preemptively prevent a great deal of discomfort by programming your mind before you drift off to sleep. Tell yourself that you will have a pleasant journey experience and wake feeling recharged, ready to face your day. It's amazing what setting the intention before an exercise will do!

Should you experience discomfort of any kind during one of the waking conscious-ness exercises, it is usually enough to simply shift your focus back to the physical body. Moving an arm or leg or even something as small as a finger or toe is often enough to bring the consciousness rushing back into the physical body. Some people experience sleep paralysis, and they lack the ability to move their arms or legs in that condition. If you struggle with this condition, start by making sure you are well rested. Sleep paralysis generally happens due to fatigue and stress. If you are not already getting between six and eight hours of sleep a night on a consistent basis, consider addressing your sleep schedule and reducing the stressful factors in your daily life before learning to lucid dream or consciously astral project.

Again, if you're afraid, it's always a good idea to preplan. Before you start doing the exercises, it might be wise to give yourself a mental command that says something like, "I am always in control of my astral projection experience, and I can return to my physical body anytime I want by simply twitching my index finger on my right hand." Something like that command is usually enough to do the trick. You will have to create the mental programming sentence that speaks to your subconscious mind. The important thing to remember is to state your intention in a positive present tense and reaffirm your control for yourself. How you do that is up to you.

There are certainly more tricks of the trade that will help the witch who is just starting out with astral projection. However, that information would take up volumes on its own. If you are interested in learning more, please see my Recommended Read-ing list at the back of this book. You'll find several really wonderful resources on this topic in there.

Astral Projection Basics

There are basically two types of astral projection—one that occurs during sleep and one that happens while awake. Everyone astral projects during sleep, but not everyone remembers their nightly travels. When we become aware of the fact that we have astral projected during sleep and we take control of the experience, it is sometimes referred to as *lucid dreaming*. In order to assist with retaining the memory of these nightly travels, some wise witches suggest keeping a dream journal on the nightstand so that we don't forget our dreams. If you struggle with journaling upon waking up, you can always use your phone's recording app to talk through the events of your dreams and transcribe the details later.

Because astral projection and sleep are so intimately connected, it is easiest to learn the skill while you sleep. Despite the added difficulty of separating the astral and physical bodies while awake, it is well worth the extra effort for witches to learn how to project during waking consciousness as well. This additional control helps witches further develop their psychic powers, which will be immensely useful in spell work, during ritual, and in countless other areas of a magickal life.

The basic technique for each stage is the same. All three stages can be done asleep or in waking consciousness. In truth, these stages are only really differentiated by the distance of the consciousness from the physical body during the projection experience. The first stage, which dislodges the astral double from the physical body, involves the physical and astral bodies still being in very close proximity to each other—often within inches. The second stage involves projecting only a small distance from the physical body. Some sources say that the distance is no more than a few feet, while other sources claim it can be as far apart as a few miles. One thing that seems consistent in all accounts is the fact that it is easier to project to familiar locations during this stage of projection. The third stage of the process involves projecting to targets at a great distance from the physical body—hundreds of miles, across oceans, and so on.

This section contains three exercises—two variations to help the witch free the astral double from the physical body and one exercise on lucid dreaming to get started with the projection experience. Should you wish to repeat your lucid dreaming experience during the waking hours, you only need to combine your chosen method of freeing the astral double from the physical form with the techniques discussed in connection to the lucid dreaming exercise. It may take some time and practice at first to translate the skill from sleeping to wakeful consciousness, but persistence is key. The dedicated witch will eventually achieve success with this practice.

To begin practicing astral projection, simply choose one of the two initial exercises in the section titled Freeing the Astral Double and master it. It doesn't matter which one you practice. They both do the same exact thing. However, some people struggle with motion sickness, and the rocking motion in the first exercise might cause them to get nauseous. Other people struggle with a fear of water, and that fear could be enough to derail their meditative experience. Choose the one that works for you, but be diligent in your practice of this exercise. It will become essential in transitioning from the lucid dreaming exercise to astral projecting in full waking consciousness.

Freeing the Astral Double

The astral body naturally falls out of alignment with the physical body during sleep, which recharges the physical body and rejuvenates the mind. This is part of why you wake up feeling refreshed and ready to face your day. However, the benefits of moving the astral and physical bodies out of alignment with each other can be reproduced at will by the witch while awake.

The keys to success when trying to make this process happen consciously are physical relaxation, willpower, and desire. The easiest way to reproduce this experience is to try projecting after a long day of performing a repetitive physical task when the body is exhausted but the mind is alert. Exhaustion can often take the place of relaxation, because both conditions weaken the body's hold on your consciousness. Think of the last time you were exhausted but your mind was still active.

Because I reside in North Carolina and my family lives in Pennsylvania, driving great distances immediately comes to mind. Though every mapping app on Earth tells me the drive should take roughly seven hours, the trip usually takes closer to ten. That's mostly because I either have to drive through Washington, DC, navigating all never-ending construction and incessant traffic, or I have to go up through the mountains, which adds roughly two more hours. After I finally reach my family home, my body is exhausted. It feels like a concerted effort just to pick up my feet or carry my bags up to my room, and when I finally fling myself onto the mattress, my body relaxes instantly, sinking into the comfortable bed my mother has lovingly prepared for me. My mind, however, does not relax. It often replays the events of the day, and I relive my journey home. I'm stuck in stop-and-go traffic again, looking at the taillights of the drivers in front of me. We barely get started moving and the driver in front of me slams on the brakes. Suddenly, I'm jolted awake. I can actually feel my body flail in the bed as if I were trying to prevent the accident.

Have you ever had a similar experience?

If so, then you have had this type of projection.

You don't have to wear yourself out just to experience astral projection in this way, though. Anything that relaxes the body but still leaves the mind active will create the proper conditions for success. A yoga practice followed by a brief period of meditation immediately comes to mind. Alternatively, you can just add either version of the exercises in this section to your regular meditation practice. If you want to find a yoga practice you can do in the privacy of your own home, there are plenty of options available in the last couple chapters of this book. You can also tune in to my Youtube channel for some guided yoga sessions designed specifically to help you with astral projection.

For your peace of mind and focus, make sure to turn off your phone, lock the doors, and set the stage for a peaceful and uninterrupted projection experience. If you have made any protections for your space or yourself, make sure they are in place before you begin. That way you can let go of all concerns regarding your health and safety. When you are ready to begin, choose one of the two exercises in this section to start on your practice. If you happen to be someone who enjoys both the rocking motion of a hammock and water, it's okay to switch between these two exercises as well. There is nothing that says you have to stick with just one of them.

Rolling Free of the Physical Body

Lie flat and relax. Close your eyes and focus on your breath for a few moments. Soon, you become aware of your body "going to sleep." Imagine that your physical body is as heavy as a bag of sand, and feel it growing heavier with each breath you take. You may even hear yourself snore. Don't worry about that. The fact that you can hear yourself snoring is proof that you are not actually asleep. You are actually listening with your subtle hearing sense. This is a good sign.

Let go of all thoughts or concerns about the world around you. Turn your mind inward instead. Become aware of an energetic body within the physical flesh. Tell yourself that this ambient energy is your astral body. Now visualize it taking on the exact shape of your physical form if it hasn't done so already. Every detail is exactly the same. The two bodies are identical in every way.

Now imagine that your physical body is just a shell or husk. Imagine that your astral body is reducing slightly in size. It shrinks evenly from all sides at once until it is encased within the physical flesh. This is not a dramatic shrinking. If the astral body shrinks a quarter inch all around, that is enough. You are merely getting the sensation that you are encased within your physical shell and noticing the slight difference between the two bodies. Again, the image of the Russian dolls comes to mind. See the astral body as one of the smaller dolls inside the stack if that visualization helps focus your mind.

Once you have become aware of the distinction between the two bodies, imagine that your astral body is gently rocking and swaying inside the stationary physical shell, as if you were lounging in a hammock, whiling away a pleasant summer afternoon. Recall the last time you relaxed in a hammock and reproduce that sensation. Feel yourself rocking from side to side. Feel the left shoulder and the left hip of the astral body crest above the lines and curves of the physical body as the right shoulder and hip descend below the surface you are lying on. Now rock the other way, feeling the right shoulder and hip rise up and protrude from the shell as the left shoulder and hip descend. Continue to sway back and forth, picking up momentum as you go.

Eventually, you may feel like you could use this momentum to roll out of and away from the physical body entirely. That is sort of the point. Allow the sensation to deepen naturally. Don't rush it.

Floating Free of the Physical Body

If you suffer from motion sickness and you have a very active imagination, that first exercise might be a little problematic for you, so use this one instead. This version came to me one night while I was taking my bath. As I was floating in the warm water, I became aware of my breathing. Then all of a sudden I noticed something that fascinated me. As I took a breath in, filling my lungs with air, my body rose up off the bottom of the tub, and I floated weightlessly in the water, bobbing up until my chest and shoulders were above the water's surface. As I exhaled, I felt my body sink, and I was placed gently back down onto the bottom of the tub again. This rising and falling action with the breath got me thinking: *That's a bit like how astral projection works!*

If you have ever experienced this sensation while taking a bath yourself, then you know exactly what feeling you are trying to reproduce. If you haven't ever paid attention to this action, it might be worth drawing yourself a bath and experiencing it for yourself. Simply relax in the bathwater, and feel your body rise up above the water's surface as you inhale. Then as you exhale, feel your body sink back beneath the water's surface and feel your back, your buttocks, and the backs of your legs touch the bottom of the tub. Pay attention to the sensation. Study it. Internalize it. This watery practice will do more for your success than anything else, because it'll make the experience real for your conscious mind.

If you like the watery floating version of this exercise better than the rolling method, use it. Follow all the steps in the rolling method until you get to the hammock visualization. Relax. Close your eyes. Let go of all thoughts or concerns regarding the outside world. Focus on coalescing your astral body within the physical form. Mold it into an exact replica in your mind's eye. Then see it shrink evenly on all sides ever so slightly before picking up with this version of the exercise.

Once you have become aware of the distinction between the two bodies, imagine that your astral body is floating inside your physical flesh. Conjure up in your mind the sensation that you experienced during your bath. Feel the front of your astral body rise gently above the surface of the physical shell. As you exhale, feel your astral body lower back beneath the surface of the physical shell. You may even feel your shoulders, buttocks, and the backs of your legs descend beneath the surface that your physical shell is lying on. That's okay. It means you're gaining momentum. That's good. Breathe in, and feel your astral form rise upward again. This time it bobs up a little further beyond the surface of the physical form. As you exhale, imagine sinking an equal distance below the surface the physical shell is resting on. Repeat the cycle of rising up on the inhale and lowering back down on the exhale until you feel yourself floating a few inches above the physical shell.

In both versions of this exercise, you may still hear sounds in the external world around you. That's okay. Again, if that happens, then you are actually hearing with your astral ears. That's a demonstration of your psychic power; acknowledge the success of that experience to yourself. You may also notice that you are able to see the ceiling above you even though your physical eyelids are shut. Again, this is proof that you have tapped into your psychic powers. Mentally acknowledge the win for yourself without allowing your excitement to bring you back into your physical body. Many witches who just start out with astral projection surprise themselves so thoroughly when one of these phenomena happen that they abruptly come crashing back into the physical world.

Lucid Dreaming

Once you have succeeded at differentiating the astral body from the physical shell and you have broken free of its pull, you are ready to project your astral double into another room of your home. Don't worry if you didn't hear with your astral ears or see with your astral eyes. Not every projection experience needs to include all five of the subtle senses. You may experience one sense or all of them. Don't judge yourself; just keep practicing until you're satisfied with your progress. The important part is that you have confidence in your ability to access these subtle senses.

Now, that you have succeeded at differentiating the astral double from the physical body, it's time to actually project yourself a short distance away from your relaxed physical shell. Under the occult principle that energy follows thought, it is actually quite easy to project to a target person, place, or thing once your astral double is separated from your physical body. You only have to do three things: Hold a clear mental picture of the target in your mind, desire to be with the target badly enough, and let go of attachment to your physical body. That's it!

If you struggle with visualization—that is, if you struggle with actually seeing images in your mind—now is the time to begin developing that skill, because the ability to conjure up an image of someone or something in its full 3D glory is essential to success at this second stage of astral projection. It works like the steering wheel of a car, directing your vehicle where to go. Remember, energy follows thought.

If you need to develop your visualization skills, start by selecting a simple object that you have around your house, something that you're already familiar with seeing. This will become your target object in your first experiments with this stage of your projection exercises. Whereas faces and complex objects are difficult for many people to reproduce imaginatively, basic shapes are easier for our minds to construct into mental pictures. For me, this object was a wooden lotus flower bowl, but it can be anything you like. Study the object with all your senses. Look at it. Notice its curves and its lines. Take stock of its general shape, but also notice any etchings, engravings, and imperfections that it might have. Feel it with your hands. Bring all your senses to bear in studying the object. Do this with your physical eyes open. Then repeat the exact same process with your eyes closed, trying to reproduce the image in your mind as you caress the object. Have fun with this part, but by the time you're done, you should absolutely know this object forward and backward, inside and out.

You must have the ability to internalize the concept of your target so deeply that it is as familiar to you as your childhood home or the fact that 2 + 2 = 4. The target must be so thoroughly entrenched within your own consciousness that you are able to bring its image up in your mind reflexively within the flash of a second. If you have to spend time building the visualization or recalling details, this next stage will be more difficult. If you still struggle with the ability to visualize after studying the object, try taking up poetry.

Poetry is the very best training for developing the mind's power of visualization. Read it, analyze it, and write some of your own. You might think painting, sculpture, photography, or some other visual medium would produce faster results, but nothing holds a candle to poetry in this regard. Adepts have long held that a study of poetry was the premiere method for developing visualization skills in a novice. This is one reason that the Druids began their training as bards.

The topic of desire doesn't need much elaboration. When you want to see the object or person badly enough, it will propel your efforts. If you don't want to see the object or person in the physical, why would you want to visit them upon the astral?

As for letting go of attachment to the physical body, the best method of doing this is to fall asleep. We release this attachment naturally each night.

Projecting in Your Sleep

As you lie down to sleep, close your eyes and focus on your breath. Slow down your breathing. Make the inhale and exhale equal in length. Do this for a few moments to relax yourself. Take your time, and don't rush the process. As we saw with the yoga pranayama or conscious breathing exercise in this book's chapter regarding the witch's elements, the breath is extremely important. Let it relax you.

When you are fully relaxed, give yourself a mental command. Something like, "I consciously project to [declare the object], and I remember my experience easily and effortlessly upon waking up." Repeat your chosen statement to yourself at least thirty times. Then conjure the image of the object in your mind's eye. As you drift off to sleep, hold the image of the target object firmly in your mind. Think of nothing else but the image and your fervent desire to be with it. This must be the last thought or concern you have before you drift off to sleep.

If you are dedicated to this practice, you will eventually come face-to-face with your target object in your dreams. The vividness of the event will rival anything you might experience during full, waking consciousness. When you have succeeded at projecting to the object in another room, choose another object a little farther away. After a few rounds of choosing objects that are farther and farther away, try projecting to a person. This person should be relatively close to your sleeping body—no more than a few miles away.

———————

Releasing attachment to the physical body while awake is often much harder for witches who are just starting out with astral projection, but it must still be done. By denying the external world and turning your consciousness inward on itself, you begin the process. However, some people need to spend a bit more attention on this part of the process than others. If you fall into that camp, try a variation on mental programming. Instead of affirming that you will remember your experience this time, replace it with something relevant to your current struggle. You can use something like, "The physical world holds no value for me right now. Nothing that happens here needs my attention. Instead, I'm going to turn inward and relax for a half an hour."

When you fully believe that nothing outside yourself is as fascinating as the internal experience, which you are currently having, combine one of the two exercises to free the astral double from the physical body with the techniques just learned. Then practice, practice, practice. You will eventually succeed at projecting during waking consciousness.

Astral Projection, Witchcraft Powers & the Siddhis

Once witches have achieved some measure of success with astral projection, they are in a prime position to begin developing the traditional psychic powers of yoga. That's because many of the traditional psychic powers associated with yoga are actually accessed through a direct awareness and control of the astral body. These powers are called *siddhis,* and it really is quite remarkable how similar their descriptions are to the psychic powers of the witch. It almost feels like the two traditions might once have been of a similar root origin.

In the Tibetan tantric yoga traditions, there was an adept named Tilopa (988–1069 CE) who made this connection abundantly clear. He founded a style of tantric yoga called *Kalachakra Tantra,* which has been translated as *Wheel of Time.* His wheel had six spokes, which were representative of six yogas. According to Ian A. Baker in his book *Tibetan Yoga,* "Tilopa's six yogas focused on inner heat, radiant bliss, clear light, lucid dreaming, transference of consciousness and navigational instructions for end of life and postmortem experiences."[119] At least three of the six yogas discussed in Tilopa's practice of tantra are directly tied to the astral body. The clear light, lucid dreaming, and transference of consciousness all have a connection to the astral body and hint at the deeper wisdom that the traditional siddhis are connected to the astral body itself.

Another translation of the word *siddhis* is *accomplishments.* In line with this translation, Patanjali does not regard these powers as magickal. Rather, he goes out of his way to talk about how ordinary these powers actually are and to show how every human being has access to them. The only thing that deprives most people of their ability to access these powers or accomplishments is distraction. In all honesty, Patanjali's approach of thinking about these powers as mundane faculties available to all of humanity probably is the best approach, because it establishes a solid foundation for success in their attainment. If they are faculties available to all of humanity, like rational thought or empathy, that knowledge can be used to bolster the witch's resolve when struggling to overcome the distraction Patanjali mentions.

In chapter 1, I mentioned that there were a great many siddhis. Different sources recount a different number. Generally speaking, most sources agree that there are eight

---

119. Ian A. Baker, *Tibetan Yoga: Principles and Practices* (Vermont: Inner Traditions, 2019), 25.

primary siddhis and then other expressions of those attainments, which stem from the original eight.

Anima

This is often described as the ability to become smaller than the smallest. In 1973, A. C. Bhaktivedanta Swami Prabhupada gave a lecture on the topic of the siddhis in London. He had this to say about this particular ability: "So a yogi, anima, he can become smaller than the smallest. We are already smaller than the smallest, because our real dimension, spiritual dimension, is one ten-thousandth part of the tip of the hair. This is our dimension. This is only outward covering, this body."[120] Swami Prabhupada is speaking directly to an audience in this lecture and making gestures to aid his communication. Imagine as you read the last two sentences of his quote that he is pointing to the world around him and gesturing to his physical body. For witches who did the phase shifting exercise in this book and felt their astral bodies growing slightly smaller than their physical bodies, the ability he is talking about here should become abundantly clear.

Mahima

This is talked about as the ability to expand one's body to an infinitely large size and translated as the *ability to become bigger than biggest* or *bigger than the universe*. For witches who are familiar with the Lesser Banishing Ritual of the Pentagram, commonly abbreviated as LBRP, this sensation will be extremely familiar.

Garima

This ability is often translated as *to become infinitely heavy* or *heavier than the heaviest*. Part of this power is to make oneself immovable by others. Yogis who attain this ability can only be moved if they choose to be moved. From the witch's elemental magick perspective, this is a version of controlling the earth elementals. Elementals exist as part of the astral plane, and, as such, the witch exerts control over them through the use of the astral body in various ways.

---

120. "Lecture BG 01.31—London," *Vanisource*, accessed February 24, 2020, https://vanisource.org/w /index.php?title=730724_-_Lecture_BG_01.31_-_London&t=hl#terms=A%E1%B9%87im%C4 %81la%E1%B9%87im%C4%81.

Laghima

This is the ability to become weightless, lighter than air, or lighter than the lightest. In addition to being the balance to garima, laghima ties directly into the astral projection exercises in this book. The ability to rise up out of the body that was experienced in the alternative phase shifting exercise calls upon this ability. When the projector buoyantly floated up above the physical sheath, that was an expression of this ability. When the projector sank back down beneath the surface of the physical body, this was a manifestation of a simplified version of garima as well.

Prapti

This attainment is often translated as *the ability to construct anything, the ability to touch the moon with one's finger, to get anything from anywhere, ability to construct anything*, and various other interpretations. In fact, of all the traditional siddhis, this one seems to have the widest variation in translation. The basic idea is that someone who has attained this siddhi can conjure up or materialize anything from anywhere at any time.

The witch's ability to conjure forth an outcome with psychism, spells, and other forms of magick certainly seems to be an outcropping of this particular talent. Some of the more fantastic examples surrounding this particular attainment talk about the immediate materialization of a desired object, like something Endora or Samantha might do on the television show *Bewitched*. However, the test questions that get asked to demonstrate what attainment of this ability might look like prove that it is not as outlandish as it may at first appear.

- Have you ever felt as if you were holding or touching something even when your hands were empty?
- Have you ever felt an itching sensation in either of your hands when there was no earthly reason for that sensation?

When people answer either of these questions in the affirmative, they are told that they are experiencing a residual echo of this attainment from a previous incarnation. These residual echoes undoubtedly belong to the astral realm. Witches and hypnotists actually have a beginner level psychic development exercise that uses the astral body in this way. Should you wish to develop your own visualization skills further and see this ability in action for yourself, you can try that exercise now and see what I mean.

Two Orbs

Hold your hands out in front of you. See that they are empty. Now close your eyes. In your mind, imagine that you are holding two orbs. One of them is a balloon with a string that is tied to your wrist. The other is a heavy orb about the weight of a bowling ball or something else that's equally heavy. Take some time to feel their different weights. Now begin describing the lightness of the balloon to yourself. In your mental voice inside your head (or out loud if you feel the need), tell yourself how light that balloon is. Talk about how it just seems to float upward, how it gently tugs on your wrist, pulling your wrist ever upward. Talk about how it just floats higher and higher. Really feel that. Then when you have felt that sensation of lightness, turn your attention to the heavy orb. Feel its weight. Feel it get heavier and heavier, dragging your arm down closer and closer to the ground. Feel your shoulder struggle to keep holding your arm up, fighting gravity. Really talk up how heavy this orb is. It just keeps getting heavier and heavier until you're nearly ready to drop it. Then switch back to the light balloon and enhance that imagery more and more in your mind. Really sense its lightness. Feel it tugging your arm up. Feel your arm rising above your shoulder. Feel that sensation in the shoulder and in your upper back. Then turn back and focus again on the heavy orb, reinforcing the heaviness imagery for yourself, truly feeling it. Keep switching back and forth between the two for a few rounds until the sensations are so palpable that you actually believe you are holding these two objects. Then open your eyes. If you've done this exercise right and really experienced the sensations, the hand attached to the balloon will be significantly higher than the hand holding the heavy orb. If you really felt the tug of the balloon or the weight of the heavy orb, then you have experienced this power in some small measure for yourself.

Prakamya

This attainment is often talked about as the ability to become whatever the practitioner desires to be. It includes fantastical and awe-inspiring powers like walking on water, flying or levitating, and even the ability to submerge oneself beneath the water and be sustained there for extended periods of time. One guru was said to live six months out of the year submerged within the Ganges. Other examples of this ability sound a bit like the witch's power of glamour. They include abilities like maintaining a youthful appearance for as long as you like and the power to become invisible at will.

Ishita

Defined as *knowing all powers and getting control over them.* However, on a practical level, the texts seem to talk about elemental powers and how to use them. A few translations talk about this power being more about having command over the forces of nature, but, again, that too seems elemental, and as has already been discussed, elementals are astral plane entities. When accounts of the witch's version of elemental magick are compared against Vedic accounts of this attainment, they seem remarkably similar.

Vashikaran

This attainment has been translated as *the ability to bring others under your control.* In the West, we have a few examples of this ability that are readily available to most witches. Commanding and compelling spells, various versions of telepathy, even hypnosis—all of these are outcroppings of this ability discussed through the lens of witchcraft, and all of them require some measure of proficiency connecting with the astral plane.

Imagine This

The waking stage of astral projection that comes after developing the ability to dream lucidly was compared to yoga's siddhis in some of the older occult texts. Many of the siddhis discussed in this chapter correspond directly to abilities of the astral body. Though many of the yoga accounts of psychic powers describe them as being manifested through the physical body, that seems more creative license than fact in most cases. There have been reputed cases where these powers have manifested on the physical plane, and I'm not discounting those cases. It certainly seems possible that some of the powers, like the ability to gain the strength of an elephant, might manifest within the physical body.[121] The classic example of this is the mother who lifts a car off her child. She is clearly manifesting this strength through the physical body. Even in the cases like the mother's loving strength, though, there is still an astral component to the physical expression of the power or ability being discussed. This is one of the many reasons why witches who desire to develop their psychic powers should learn to astral project.

---

121. Stiles, *Yoga Sutras*, 37 (III, 25).

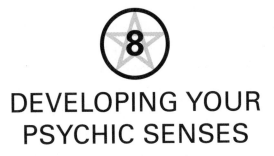

DEVELOPING YOUR
PSYCHIC SENSES

When most people think of developing their psychic talents, their second sight is the first skill they try to tackle. It just seems to be the skill that everyone focuses on when they think about psychic powers. It's the most flashy of the subtle senses, and it is also the most effective at alleviating doubts when nothing else will. Generally speaking, most people are visual. Even witches, who primarily experience the subtle realms through their other senses, have a tendency to use visual language when talking about the occult. They talk about things like *seeing the circle* or *seeing spirits*. People just naturally seem to talk in terms of sight, even when they're talking about nonphysical reality. For example, phrases like "I see what you're saying," "I see your point," or simply "I see" are all used in place of "I understand."

The focus on the second sight above the other subtle senses can actually be quite problematic for many witches. Their inability to see the subtle realms of reality can often be crushing to a new witch's ego. When they fail to see psychically at first, they imagine that they aren't psychic. They tell themselves that they just don't have "the gift." In some cases, this particular obstacle can even turn these budding witches away from their magickal paths entirely. It's all rather unfortunate and so unnecessary.

The focus on second sight over the other psychic senses was a huge problem for me personally when I started out in witchcraft. My own natural psychic abilities were more intuitive than visual. My intuition is so strong, in fact, that it often blocked my visual psychic experiences in the past. I always got information when I would do the psychic exercises in Wicca 101 books, but I never saw what the author described in the exercise. Instead, I would get faint impressions, an intuitive understanding, or a feeling connected to the exercise in question. For the longest time, I thought I was third eye blind or that I was in some other way deficient.

As frustrating as that experience was, my self-doubt never made me give up on my witchcraft. In fact, it actually made me work harder as a witch. Remember earlier when I said that I'm like a dog with a bone? This is what I mean. Ever since I can remember, I had wanted to be a witch, and, in my mind, a witch was psychic. What's more, I bought into the idea that a psychic must be clairvoyant. That's all there was to it. There really wasn't any room for debate as far as I was concerned. If you were a witch, you were clairvoyant. So, as all the gods were my witness, I was going to become psychic or die trying, because there was no way in Hel that I wasn't going to be a witch!

It wasn't until I watched Tim Burton's *Sleepy Hollow* that I fully appreciated my intuition. My moment of revelation came after the Horseman barged into the midwife's house and collected the heads of both husband and wife. As the Horseman was getting ready to leave the cottage, he sensed that there was someone else there. He stopped abruptly before leaving the cottage, turned back around and then immediately went over to the exact spot in the cottage where the midwife's child lay hidden beneath the floorboards to deliver the fatal blow to the last surviving member of the Killian family. The Horseman was intuitive!

For the first time, I saw how psychic intuition could be an incredibly useful skill. Never mind that the Horseman is the villain or that several fictional people had to lose their heads because of his psychic proficiency with this skill that I devalued so easily. That seemed like a small price to pay for my revelation. Intuition no longer seemed like a consolation prize for failing to see psychically. It now felt powerful and even glamorous. It was something I could be proud of in my witchy bag of tricks. Thank you, Mr. Burton!

Two things helped me overcome my own obstacles.

First, I recognized what I told you earlier: the psychic senses are actually just astral senses. We all have all of them. If we didn't, we wouldn't be able to have their physical plane counterparts. The subtle sense of sight connected to the astral body is often called *clairvoyance* by many psychics and witches. The prefix *clair-* means *clear*. So the term *clairvoyance* applied to the astral body's subtle sense of sight means *clear vision*. The other subtle senses get similarly labeled. Clairaudience, which means *clear hearing*, is the subtle sense of hearing connected to the astral body. Clairsentience, which means *clear feeling*, is the astral body's sense of feeling. Clairalience, which means *clear smelling*, is the astral sense of smell, and clairgustance, which means *clear tasting*, is the astral sense of taste.

The second thing that helped me was my moment of cinematic humility. When I finally gave in to my natural strength and I began exploring my astral senses through the lens of my intuition, I started to see success with my psychic development. Eventually, that success even began to strengthen my clairvoyance.

These two realizations turbocharged my progress, and they can help you, too. Don't write your own psychic strengths off just because one of the other abilities seems flashier or more powerful to you. If you are diligent in your efforts and if you learn to translate your successes from your strengths toward helping you overcome the areas where you struggle, you will be able to develop all five subtle senses effectively.

While all five subtle senses are equally valuable, clairalience and clairgustance tend to come naturally after the other three psychic senses are fully engaged. That said, the order in which you focus on the other three is irrelevant. Feel free to jump to the one you're strongest with and get a fast win under your belt or do them in the order provided.

Here is a simple universal fluid condenser. Use it to develop your subtle senses or when casting elemental spells. It will greatly boost your efforts.

Making a Universal Fluid Condenser

Take a handful of dried chamomile flowers and place them in a pot. Cover the herbs with cold water. Then put the lid on the pot, and let it boil for approximately twenty minutes. Let it cool with the lid on. Once it is completely cool, filter the herbs out, pouring the chamomile concoction into a clean pot. Reduce it to about ¼ cup with the lid on. After it cools, mix it with equal amounts of alcohol to preserve the chamomile extract. Then add approximately ten drops of gold tincture. Shake well before each use.

Clairsentience

As I hope my story about Tim Burton's Headless Horseman demonstrated, clairsentience is actually quite powerful. What I don't think I have yet managed to communicate, though, is just how powerful and just how all-encompassing this particular psychic ability truly is. A common example of clairsentience in action involves ghost hunters. We're all familiar with the people who seek out and explore haunted places. Ghost hunters often describe the sensation of someone breathing on the backs of their necks in a dark room. However, clairsentience is not just the ability to feel psychically, like the tactile sensations experienced through our physical bodies. There are much more profound expressions of this truly remarkable psychic sense for us to consider. For example, that eerie feeling of being watched by a presence that isn't objectively there, which some people have described in haunted houses, is an impalpable form of clairsentience.

Once you have begun to tap into your own subtle sense of clairsentience, you will greatly improve your empathy and intuition. They are both merely higher forms of clairsentience. As you become more adept at feeling on the subtle levels, you will also improve your skills with psychometry and the materialization of thoughts and beings, like thoughtforms, spirits, or the elemental servitors of the grimoires. All these powers and more have their origins within the subtle sense of clairsentience. In truth, it really is an incredibly powerful skill, and, just like physical touch helps us navigate the world we live in, clairsentience helps us navigate the subtle realms.

Activating Your Clairsentience

When you are ready to begin your training in clairsentience, you can employ the use of the universal fluid condenser that you just made. Shake the fluid condenser to mix it back up, then add roughly ten drops to a bottle of carrier oil of your choosing, and because you'll also have to shake the oil after you put the fluid condenser in, make sure the bottle has a tight-fitting lid. Good options are jojoba, or, if you plan on using it all relatively quickly, olive oil or grape-seed oil will do the trick.

Pour a small amount of the oil into the palm of your hand. As you rub your hands together, imagine that the element of water exists all around you. Remember that elemental water is cold and constricting. If you are someone who has a fear of water, just work with those two qualities. If you're someone who loves the water, you can choose to add in the component of moisture as well—either way is fine. Breathe in some of that elemental water energy. Feel your hands grow cold and tight (and wet) as you engage the element of water with your imaginative will. Then anoint your forehead, your torso, and your hands and thighs with the oil.

Lie down in a comfortable position and close your eyes. If you like the water, imagine that you are floating in the tub once again, like you did when you freed your astral double from the physical shell of your body in the last chapter. If you fear the water, simply change the visualization. Instead, imagine that you are surrounded by a cool or cold energy that caresses your body.

Feel yourself rise and fall, cresting above the water's surface as you inhale. Then notice how you sink back beneath the water's edge as you exhale. Continue with this pleasant sensation of bobbing up and down as you float in the bathtub. Allow yourself to relax there, knowing that you are completely safe and secure. Allow the idea of the tub to slip from your mind and instead just allow yourself to float aimlessly on the elemental water.

Transfer your consciousness to your solar plexus. To do this, simply think of the energy center and the corresponding region of the physical body. See or feel it light up in the astral body if that helps. Allow yourself to float on the elemental water with your mind operating from within your solar plexus. Take stock of any shifts or changes within yourself. Are you able to get a better feel for things?

When your consciousness is firmly seated in your solar plexus, imagine that the magnetic ability of water transfers into you. Breathe it in. Feel the cool moist energy enter your nose and travel to your lungs. Feel the pores of your body open up to take in more of this primal universal energy. Imagine it enlivening every particle of your being as it awakens your clairsentience.

Notice how the magnetic energy seems to be collecting in your solar plexus. Allow the energy to rush in, filling up the energy center before moving up into the heart. Feel the water fill the heart chakra, just as it did the solar plexus. Then repeat the process for all the places you anointed with the fluid condenser—the third eye, the hands, and the thighs. As you get better at this exercise, try splitting your consciousness and feeling it in two places at once. When this happens, simultaneously magnetize both of your hands with the element of water. Then repeat the process with your thighs. Until then, it's okay to focus on one limb at a time.

Once you are thoroughly convinced that you have awoken your clairsentience, then release the concept of magnetism from your body back into the elemental water that surrounds you. To do this, simply empty your mind as you inhale, and as you exhale, think about releasing the magnetic powers of water back to where they came from. Feel that infinite expanse of water transform back into your bathwater again, allowing yourself to float there in the tub for a while. Then when you are ready to come out of your meditation, open the tub's drain and feel the water gradually dissolving away from your body, going back into the ether from whence it came.

Open your eyes, and readjust to your surroundings.

Now that you have a universal fluid condenser and this basic exercise for unlocking your clairsentient potential, you may use them whenever you have need of them. In the beginning, you may need the condenser and the exercise quite often. You should endeavor to memorize the steps of the exercise so that they become second nature to you. Over time, as you become more confident in your own clairsentient abilities, you may also find that you don't need them as much, or at all. Ideally, your clairsentience will just seem to turn on at will or when it is needed.

A Yoga Sequence for Clairsentience

However, should you still be struggling to develop your clairsentient potential, here is a basic yoga sequence that will help you tap into the power. It is not essential that you do these exercises to tap into your clairsentience. However, if you are struggling to achieve results with the previous exercise alone, this sequence may just be enough to tip the scale in your favor.

This sequence is slow and peaceful, because it is meant to keep you cool and relaxed, like the water element. So, breathe and move slowly. Hold each pose for anywhere from two to ten minutes and allow the stretch to deepen over time. Do not force it. Don't struggle. Instead, just be present in the moment and allow your practice to be whatever it is in that moment.

Child's Pose

The clairsentient yoga practice begins with a focus on softening the heart. To do this, simply hold child's pose for at least two minutes. To get into child's pose, start by getting on your hands and knees. Spread your knees wide apart (maybe even a little wider than hip distance if you can manage it), and, if possible, keep your big toes touching. Sit straight up. Imagine that the crown of your head is attached to a balloon and that the balloon is pulling you up, lengthening your spine. Then as you exhale, fold forward, hinging from the hips. Bring your third eye toward the mat. If you can't get your head to touch the mat, you may use a pillow or a block to rest your head on so that you are comfortable. Your arms may either be out in front of you, reaching for the edge of your mat, or held by your sides with your hands back by your feet. Both are equally beneficial, and you may want to switch it up between practice sessions.

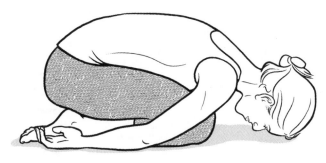

Child's Pose

Sphinx

After about two minutes, inhale yourself back up from child's pose onto all fours with your shoulders stacked above your wrists and your hips above your knees. Straighten out the knees; rest your thighs, shins, and the tops of your feet on the ground. Then exhale yourself gently down onto the mat so that your stomach presses firmly against the earth, like you're lowering yourself back down to the ground after doing an assisted push-up. Lower onto your forearms, stacking the elbows directly under the shoulders. As you inhale, press your forearms into the mat, and lift your chest and head up, keeping your chin parallel to the ground. Imagine yourself like a child watching Saturday morning cartoons. It should look very much like the Egyptian Sphinx, which is where this pose gets its name. Mimic the statue. Hold for five minutes. If you struggle to keep this pose for that long, start with a practice of ten slow, deep belly breaths and work your way up to the full five minutes.

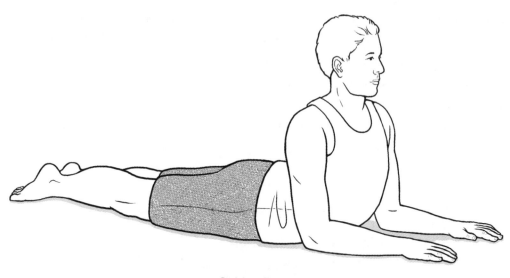

Sphinx Pose

Windshield Wiper Pose

Transition onto your back. Stretch your arms out at shoulder height. Place your feet flat on the floor and your knees together. Take slow, deep belly breaths, making sure to pull your belly button all the way in toward your spine with each exhalation. Gently lower your knees to the right side and look over your left shoulder. Then lower your knees to the left side and look over your right shoulder. Raise and lower your legs in line with your breath, exhaling the legs down to either side and inhaling them back up to center. Repeat for two minutes, paying attention to both sides of the motion equally.

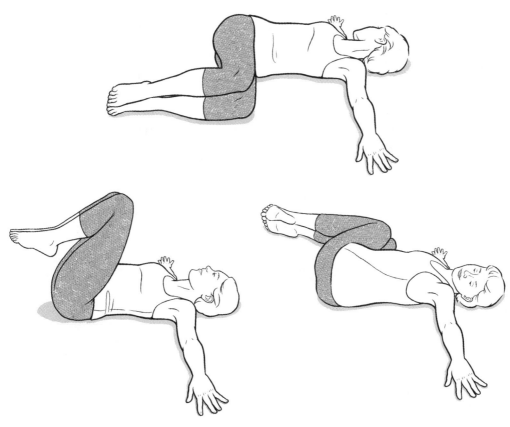

Windshield Wiper Pose

Happy Baby

The next time you inhale your legs up to center, stop the windshield wiper action. Take another exhale with your feet on the floor and your knees pointing toward the sky. Inhale your knees up toward your chest and open them slightly wider than torso width apart. Reach up and grab hold of your feet, bringing your knees closer to your armpits. Stack the ankles above the knees so that your shins are perpendicular to the floor. Push the heels up toward the ceiling as you press the soles of your feet into your hands or a strap wrapped around the feet as you pull down to create resistance. Hold for two or three minutes.

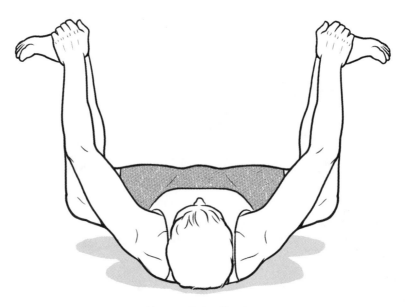

Happy Baby Pose

Savasana

Release your feet and allow your legs to lower gently onto the mat. Let your arms fall by your sides with your palms facing upward. Close your eyes, and pick up with the Activating Your Clairsentience exercise. If you need the fluid condenser to help you achieve this altered state of consciousness, apply it to the specified areas before fully relaxing into your savasana position. Hold this posture for the length of the clairsentient meditation, and follow the instructions as written. (If you need to use the universal fluid condenser infused oil, put it on before sinking into this pose.)

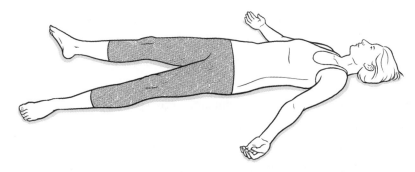

Corpse Pose

Clairaudience

Like clairsentience, clairaudience should not be undervalued. We often take for granted how much of our sensory information about our surroundings comes to us through our sense of hearing. Hearing your name called by a voice on the wind while drifting between the sleeping and wakeful states is often a very cathartic moment, especially after a loved one has crossed beyond the veil. Hearing a disembodied voice when ghost hunting can be just as thrilling as seeing an apparition. However, it's important to point out that clairaudience is not just the ability to hear things psychically. It also includes the ability to understand the things you hear, which is in and of itself a bit impressive. For example, did it ever seem odd to you that psychics who had developed their clairaudience were able to understand spirits who didn't speak their own language?

At first, this ability starts in a rather mundane way. It begins as hearing your own internal mental voice. There are people who struggle with hearing any voice at all in their heads. Their thoughts are amorphous and general. They don't think in cohesive sentences, but rather in the abstract. There are others who think only in pictures. For those people, clairaudience is a bit more difficult, though certainly not impossible, to develop.

In order to develop this talent, it is merely a matter of these abstract thinkers forcing themselves to change their thought patterns. It starts with them talking their way through their thoughts out loud until their minds begin concretizing those thoughts and thinking in complete sentences automatically, saying something like, "I am currently seeing an image of a red ball in my mind." After the mind has started to associate thinking with the verbal word, the abstract thinker can begin thinking in complete sentences without the physical anchor of speaking. Most importantly, the abstract thinker must turn their mind away from focusing on mental images during practice sessions where they are trying to develop this talent.

Physically, stronger muscles have a tendency to compensate for weaker ones. In psychic training, stronger talents tend to overshadow weaker or underdeveloped ones, like my clairsentience did with my clairvoyance. For those who have the will to force themselves not to rely on their strengths but focus on their weaknesses instead, this process can move very quickly. For those who rely on their strengths unknowingly or who can't force their mind to abandon old habits, this process can take significantly longer. The more you are able to exercise self-control, the easier this process goes.

After you have gained the ability to think in your own internal voice, you will eventually be able to hear the thoughts of others. Generally, these thoughts will present through your voice and your perspective. For example, if someone wants a bite of chocolate, you might hear the phrase "I want chocolate" in your own voice and feel like you are the one who actually wants the chocolate, even if you don't personally like chocolate yourself. If you hear other voices, please talk to the appropriate mental health professional. Hearing voices other than your own is not usually part of clairaudience. It can actually be quite problematic. If you do happen to hear voices other than your own internal mental voice, do not judge yourself. You've done nothing wrong, and you have nothing to be ashamed of, but you do need to speak with a qualified licensed mental health professional who can help you navigate the situation appropriately.

Activating Your Clairaudience

All sound travels on the air. Without the influence of the air element, we could shout at the top of our lungs and nobody would hear a word we said. This fact is just as true within the psychic worlds as it is in the physical world. So, our clairaudient exercises take this principle as their foundation.

After you have moistened your cotton balls with the oil infused with about ten drops of universal fluid condenser, squeeze the cotton balls. You don't want them dripping into your ears. You just want a little bit of the mixture. If you have ear pain, you have had ear surgery, or you have a tear in your eardrum, don't put anything in the ears without talking to a qualified medical professional first.

Find a comfortable seated position, either on the floor or in a straight-backed chair, and slow down your breathing. Make the inhale and exhale equal in length. Imagine that your entire body fills up like a balloon as you breathe in. See yourself taking in the element of air. Empty your mind and think of nothing as you exhale. Then resume your visualization again as you take in the next breath. You want to start with no more than seven breaths. (You can build up to accumulating more of the air element within you as you get more advanced in your practice, but in the beginning, stick to seven breaths.) Think to yourself in that still small voice in your head, "Like calls unto like. This elemental air within carries the quality of clairaudience to my astral ears." When you are certain that the air element within you is fully imbued with your imaginative wish for clairaudience, exhale the elemental air into the cotton balls.

As long as your ears are healthy, put the cotton balls in so that they stay in place without you having to hold them. Now, close your eyes again. Imagine that you have become clairaudient. Think about what that would be like. Start by talking this out verbally while repeating your words in your mental voice in your head as you do so. Then, as time goes by and you get better at the exercise, try just using your mental voice alone. Keep focusing on transmuting your thoughts into words and learning to differentiate your internal voice from the psychic din that permeates everything. Imagine that the cotton balls soaked in elemental air have yet a more subtle element within them, and this element is calling forth the gift of clairaudience. This element is ether, or what some occult texts refer to as the *etheric principle*. It is cold, light, and immovable. Imagine that the ether is the color indigo, and see your ears become that color. As they do, you feel a gentle coolness take hold, very much like the tingling sensation you receive from using eucalyptus oil on the skin. Suddenly your ears feel lighter as a gentle breeze moves through the cotton balls, caressing your ears and activating your own clairaudience as it does.

Meditate on the ether's influence for a while, focusing first on hearing your own thoughts. Then, as your meditation practice grows, focus on differentiating your thoughts from errant thoughts floating on the ether.

When you are ready to come out of this meditation, dissolve the etheric principle. See the indigo color get absorbed by the cotton balls. Feel the cool, tingling sensation calm as the ether leaves your ears and moves back into the elemental air. Let this all be absorbed into the cotton balls. Emerge from your trance slowly, and then remove the cotton balls from your ears. As time goes on and your clairaudient meditations become stronger, you will not need the cotton balls or the universal fluid condenser. Instead, all you will need to do is imagine the etheric principle entering your ears and enlivening your clairaudience, but just like learning to ride a bike, the training wheels help bring about faster success.

———————

Just like the clairsentient exercises, you will not need to do these exercises forever. You will eventually internalize the process, and your clairaudience will respond whenever you will it to or when you have need of it. However, in the beginning, you may need some extra help tapping into it. If this exercise was not enough, try the following yoga sequence to kick things into high gear.

A Yoga Sequence for Clairaudience

As with clairsentience, yoga can help you develop your astral sense of hearing. While most people in the West associate yoga with flexibility, strength, and working out, those are not its only benefits. Yoga has also been known to increase circulation, promote nerve functionality, relax muscle tissue, and so much more—all of which are helpful with maintaining a healthy sense of hearing. This yoga sequence is designed to increase the circulation of blood into the physical ears, align the astral body with the physical body so that the psychic sense of hearing can be engaged, and release tension in the neck so that you can relax enough to engage your clairaudience. During your resting meditation at the end of this sequence, plug in the previous exercise on activating your clairaudience and repeat it just as you did before.

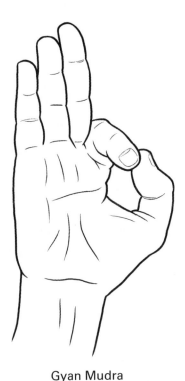

Gyan Mudra

For the first three exercises, you will be holding your hands in the Gyan mudra to engage the subtle energies of the astral body. This is the famous hand gesture that everyone always associates with yoga. Its purpose is to increase concentration and mental clarity. To begin this mudra, place your hands on your thighs in a simple seated position with your legs crossed in front of you. Then simply bend the index fingers and the thumbs on each hand so that the touch. Keep the other three fingers on each hand together and outstretched. That's it. It's really that simple. This mudra regulates air within the body.

Head Rotations

Imagine that you are shaking your head no. Now slow it down, and pair it up with your breath. As you exhale, look over your left shoulder. Then inhale back to center. Exhale to look over your right shoulder. Then repeat the inhale, bringing your head back to center. Do fifteen to twenty rotations.

Neck Flexion & Extension

Now imagine that you are nodding your head yes, but slow it down to be in line with your breath in the same way that you did with the previous exercise. Lower your chin to your chest as you exhale. Inhale your chin up to the sky. Make sure to take the full length of the inhalation and exhalation to transition the chin from one position to the next. Repeat fifteen to twenty times in all.

Neck Rolls

Bring your head back to neutral with your chin parallel to the floor. On your next exhale, lower your chin back down to your chest. Inhale and roll your head up across your chest, bringing your right ear close to your right shoulder. Continue to revolve the head upward until your chin is pointing up to the sky as you finish your inhale. As you begin to exhale, roll your head back down in an arch on the other side. First, bring your left ear close to your left shoulder. Then return your chin back down toward your chest. Continue rolling your head in line with your breath in this manner for ten to twelve full rotations. Then switch directions and complete the exercise by performing the same number of rotations the other way.

Downward Dog Pose

Release your hands from your mudra position. Lean forward over your thighs and place your palms flat on the ground in front of you. This may raise your tailbone off the mat. If not, keep leaning forward until it does. Then pivot over the knees and work your way into a tabletop position with your hands under your shoulders and your knees under your hips. (Alternatively, you can get into this position in any way that feels comfortable for you. Don't get hung up on the transition. It's the pose we're after here.) Once you are in your tabletop position, gently lift your knees up off the ground by pressing your hands and toes into the mat. Concentrate on pulling your tailbone up toward the sky. If you need to, imagine that a balloon has been tied to the end of your tailbone, and it is gently tugging you upward, bending you at the hips, lengthening the legs, and stretching the arms. Push your thighs backward and straighten your knees as much as you feel comfortable without locking them. Now take five to ten slow, deep breaths with your eyes closed.

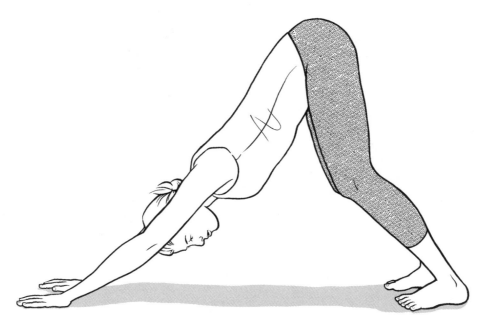

Downward-Facing Dog Pose

Legs up the Wall Pose

When you are ready to finish your yoga practice for clairaudience, go ahead and make your way onto your back. Find a comfortable position near a wall, and stretch your legs up the wall, bringing your sit bones as close to the wall as you can get them. Ideally, your glutes will be pressed firmly up against the wall, and your heels, calves, and the backs of your thighs will be touching the wall. Once you are comfortable, close your eyes and let your mind turn inward. Turn your thoughts back to the Activating Your Clairaudience exercise from earlier in this chapter, and try it again.

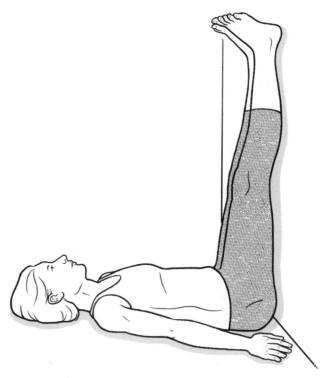

Legs up the Wall Pose

Clairvoyance

I just love the way that Mat Auryn, witch and author of the book *Psychic Witch*, talks about clairvoyance. In that book, he divides clairvoyance up between internal and external expressions of the power. He says, "Internal clairvoyance is the ability to see something on the screen of your mind. Internal clairvoyance is experienced with symbolism and visions. External clairvoyance is the ability to see an overlay of vision over your regular sensory sight."[122]

122. Mat Auryn, *Psychic Witch: A Metaphysical Guide to Meditation, Magick & Manifestation* (Woodbury, MN: Llewellyn, 2020), 56.

What Auryn calls *internal clairvoyance*, I have always referred to as *visualization*. Witches do not have to develop their clairvoyance to the point of seeing the "overlay of vision over your regular sensory sight" in order to be effective psychically. Normal visualization techniques are often enough to achieve magickal success. However, if a witch diligently practices the following exercises, it is certainly possible to develop the external version of clairvoyance.

Activating Your Clairvoyance

When we talk about clairvoyance, we are really dealing with two separate things. First, we are talking about aligning the astral body with the physical body in such a way that the two sets of eyes line up. Imagine it like your astral eyes are looking through your physical eyes, enhancing the quality of your vision. However, proper alignment is not enough. We are also talking about working with the element of fire through the aspect of light. Without illuminating the field of vision, there are no images to see. Everything remains cloaked in darkness, and we see only blackness. This is just as true in the subtle realms as it is in the physical realms. This exercise aligns the astral and physical bodies and then illuminates the astral eyes so that you can awaken your subtle vision.

Instead of using the fluid condenser for this exercise, pour boiling water over equal parts chamomile and eyebright. You only really need a cup. Soak two cotton balls in the infusion after it cools. Squeeze any excess moisture from the cotton, and then see yourself surrounded by elemental fire. Feel it all around you. Its attributes are expansion and heat. As you breathe in, imagine that you are taking the elemental fire into your body. As you exhale, breathe that elemental fire out onto the cotton balls. See the fire leave your body as light, and see the cotton balls become so absorbed with elemental fire that they practically glow. Again, it's enough to merely visualize this. You do not have to experience the overlay of vision that Auryn talks about. Then lie down flat, close your eyes, and place the cotton balls over your closed eyelids. Imagine two brilliant suns shining brightly against your closed eyelids.

To get the astral body to align with the physical body, go back to the first astral projection exercise from the last chapter, the exercise where you practiced rolling back and forth inside your body. If you did the floating version, you can use that here, too. Simply eliminate the watery imagery from your visualization. Allow yourself to experience that sensation again, but, this time, consciously slow the rocking or floating until you are able to make minor adjustments to fit your astral body within the lines and contours of your physical body. It's important that you visualize the astral body forming into an exact replica of the physical body for this exercise. See it coalesce as the astral double. Take your time imagining the two bodies lining up perfectly. Some people who naturally have astral sight claim that the astral plain has a blue-gray hazy color, like gun smoke. Clairvoyants also claim that this is true of the astral body. If using the color imagery helps you gain control over the astral body, see the astral body as a pale blue-gray body of light, and visualize that blue-gray set of eyes permeating every cell of your physical eyeballs.

Once your astral and physical eyes have aligned, turn your attention back to the elemental fire energy. Feel the expansive heat all around you. See that elemental fire convert to astral light. Visualize the astral light in your mind's eye as identical to natural sunlight. As you inhale, begin breathing that astral light into your body. Breathe it in through your nose into your lungs, but also breathe it in through every pore on your body. Let the light caress your skin and then let your skin soak it up, like a sponge soaks up water. Feel your body becoming "saturated" with this radiant astral light. To do this, simply breathe in and say, "I absorb universal light into my body," as you imagine yourself soaking it up. As you exhale, let all thoughts leave your mind. Think of absolutely nothing until you begin inhaling again, and then repeat your mantra ("I absorb universal light into my body").

Once you have filled your astral body with the radiant, white astral light and you are like a saturated sponge, use the power of your imagination and concentration to impregnate the light in your body with the quality of clairvoyance. Tell the light "You are now the very essence of clairvoyance" with that still small mental voice you hear inside your mind. As you program the light, become aware that this light sees everything. It has shone upon everything at one time or another. It penetrates everything eventually. Neither space nor time pose an obstacle to the light you have just accumulated within your body.

Once you have finished accumulating this universal light and programmed it for your intended purpose, feel it pressing against the edges of your astral body. Feel the dynamic state of tension it produces within you. Visualize it radiating out of you in all directions. Now imagine that the light begins to move away from the farthest reaches of your body, starting with your fingers and toes. Visualize it moving toward the center of your body, up to your head, and finally accumulating in your eyes, as if it were pooling there. Visualize your eyes (both your astral eyes and your physical eyes) glowing with this radiant universal light.

Allow yourself to practice this exercise for at least ten minutes at a time in the beginning. As time goes by and you become more adept at imagining this scenario, you can extend the time limit for each practice session incrementally. However, it is extremely important that when you are finished with your session, you release the astral light back to the ether from whence it came and that you stop consciously aligning your physical and astral bodies. To release the light, see it leave the eyes, moving back into the head, spreading back out through the rest of the body, back toward your extremities, until your entire astral body is radiating, practically glowing, with that light once again. Then as you exhale, think to yourself, "I release the astral light back to its source," as you imagine it leaving your body. This time, as you inhale, empty your mind. Think of nothing until you start exhaling again, and then repeat your mantra in your mental voice. It's exactly the opposite of what you did to accumulate the light. It's just done in reverse.

Now, allow yourself to take a few moments and release the control over the astral body. Simply stop willing it to align perfectly with your physical body. Release the idea that it is an exact replica of your physical body. Allow it to shift back into its natural state. If it stays there for a while, don't worry. It will eventually ebb and flow or move according to what is natural for it. Simply turn your mind to other things and let all thoughts of your astral body disappear from your mind.

Instead, simply focus on your breath. Take seven to ten slow, deep belly breaths and tell yourself that you are ready to come back to the mundane world. Tell yourself that you are fully awake and you feel refreshed from your exercise, and then, when you are ready, open your physical eyes and go about the events of your day.

A Yoga Sequence for Clairvoyance

This yoga sequence is designed to build heat in the body, since fire is the element most associated with clairvoyance. This yoga sequence is designed for witches who are completely new to yoga. If you are already taking yoga classes at a studio, you may want to ask your teacher for more intense ways to build heat using yoga. However, for the purposes of this book, I wanted to give you something that almost anyone could do in the privacy of their own home. The goal is to get your body moving and produce a little heat before relaxing you for a meditation. You might sweat. If you do, take that as a sign that you have been successful at tapping into the fire element. If you don't sweat, do not let that discourage you. You don't need to generate that much heat in order for this exercise to work. All you need is the warm sensation so that your mind can tap into it in your savasana at the end. Whatever your body does during this particular yoga practice will be okay as long as when you lie down for your savasana (corpse pose) meditation at the end of it, your body is a little tired and your mind is active.

During your resting meditation at the end of this sequence, plug in the previous exercise on activating your clairvoyance through the universal light meditation and repeat it just as you did before.

Hero Pose

Start in hero pose by kneeling on your mat with your knees together and your thighs parallel to the floor. Separate your feet slightly wider than hip distance apart. Lay the tops of your feet against the mat with your toes pointing straight back behind you and lean slightly forward into your thighs. Take several deep belly breaths here. Focus on making your inhale and exhale equal in length. As you inhale, allow your belly to extend out, like a cauldron. As you exhale, pull your belly button in, imagining that you are trying to press it up against you spine. Then repeat the process two or three more times.

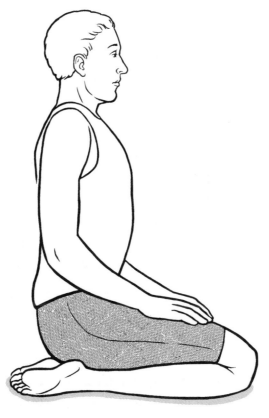

Hero Pose

Tabletop Pose

On your next inhale, lean forward and place your palms on the ground in front of you, pivoting into a tabletop position with your shoulders stacked above your elbows, which are stacked above your wrists. Your hands should be shoulder distance apart. This should also bring your hips into proper alignment, stacking them above your knees. Your knees should be hip distance apart.

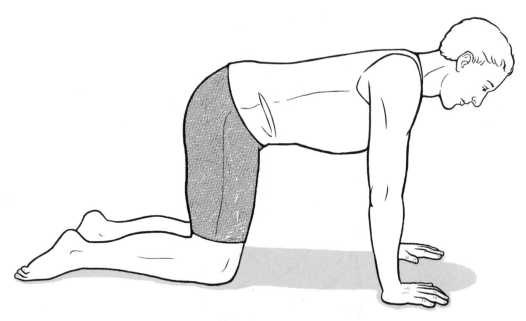

Tabletop Pose

Cat-Cow Pose

On the inhalation, as your belly begins to fill with air (reproduce that imagery of the cauldron), imagine that your back is curved like the inside surface of the cauldron. Imagine that someone could hold water in the concave depression this motion creates in the small curve of your back. As you exhale, pull your belly button in close to your spine and arch your back, like a cat that has just been scared. This pose is called *cat-cow*, because, as I just described, the exhalation looks like a frightened cat and the inhalation looks like your belly is mimicking a cow's udders. Repeat this motion, moving with the breath, creating a controlled wavelike motion, inhaling cow, exhaling cat, for ten to fifteen breaths.

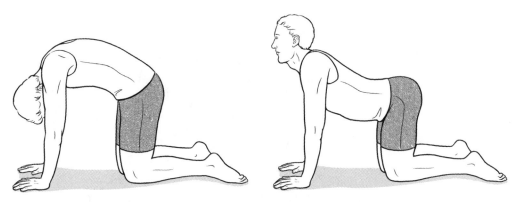

Cat-Cow Pose

Downward-Facing Dog Pose

Move your hands slightly forward from your shoulders. Spread your fingers as you press your palms into the mat, and curl your toes under, stretching out the soles of your feet. As you exhale, lift your knees up off the floor slightly, and press your sit bones up to the ceiling and backward at the same time, lengthening your legs as you do so. You do not have to straighten your legs or lock your knees. In fact, it is better that you do not lock your knees. (Make sure to leave a slight bend in your knees even in the most extreme versions of this pose.) Hold this pose for ten to fifteen breaths. The slower you cycle through your breathing while in this pose, the longer you'll hold it, and the more heat you'll build.

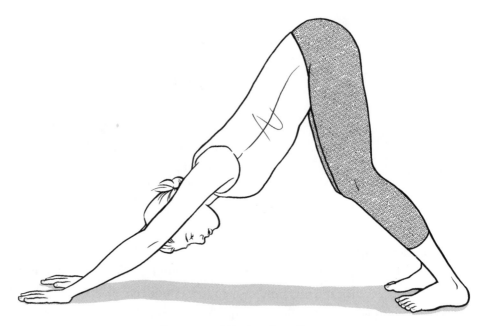

Downward-Facing Dog Pose

Return to tabletop by bending the knees and pivoting forward so that your knees come directly under your hips and bring your hands back underneath your shoulders. Knees should again be hip distance apart and hands should be shoulder distance apart on the mat beneath you.

Child's Pose

Bring your big toes together and sit back on your heels, much like you did in hero pose earlier (but this time your toes are touching each other). Separate your knees hip distance apart, if they are not already in that position. As you exhale, lower your torso toward the ground so that it rests upon your thighs. Push your tailbone backward as you press the crown of your head toward the front of the room, creating dynamic tension along the length of your back. Imagine that two forces are playing tug-of-war with you, one trying to pull you forward, the other trying to pull you back. Lay your palms on the mat with your arms outstretched in front of you, reaching for the edge of the mat. Take fifteen to thirty slow, deep belly breaths here.

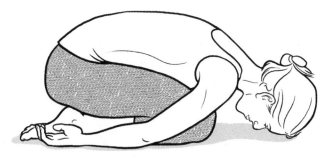

Child's Pose

Savasana

After you are done with your child's pose, go ahead and reposition yourself supine on the ground, with your back pressed firmly against the mat. Feel the back of your head, your shoulder blades, your back, your glutes, the backs of your thighs, your calves, and your heels all supported by the earth beneath you. Allow your arms to fall by your side, palms facing up toward the sky, and then let go of all conscious control of your body. Just observe it for a moment. Now, when you are ready, turn your thoughts back to the Activating Your Clairvoyance exercise from earlier in this chapter, and try it again.

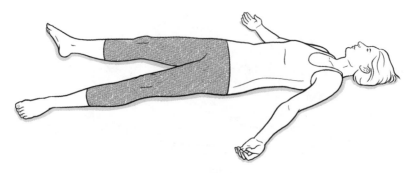

Corpse Pose

Making Sense of Psychic Phenomena

Hopefully, the astral body's role in helping witches tap into their innate psychic ability has become more clear by this point. All people have access to these powers. Sometimes it just takes a little time and practice to unlock them. Understanding the astral body's role in tapping into these abilities will make it easier to succeed at developing these abilities.

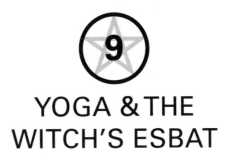

YOGA & THE
WITCH'S ESBAT

This is where the magick happens!

While it seems common practice today for witches to work magick whenever they get together, this wasn't always the way. In my own line of witchcraft, we generally didn't work magick at the sabbats unless there was a dire emergency, which might have included someone in the coven needing us to work a healing for them or a loved one. The sabbats were reserved as a time to connect with the seasonal cycles and to recharge our energetic batteries. Instead, we tended to save our general magickal workings for the Esbats, where we could focus exclusively on the intention of the spell to be worked that night.

The word *Esbat* "is held and claimed as a gathering 'to frolick', from the old French. Such a meaning should give a hint as to what witches would do at an Esbat."[123] Gardner's quote about releasing the power from a witch's body, mentioned in chapter 2, hints at this same mirth and pleasure. Through various acts of ecstasy, witches are able to raise and direct power toward the intended purpose of the Esbat ritual.

---

123. Tarostar, *The Sacred Pentagraph: Books IV & V* (Cincinnati: Left Hand Press, 2019), 14.

The Moon

While the sun is the source of life on Earth and it reigns supreme in the Wheel of the Year, the moon holds sway over the witch's Esbat. As the closest heavenly body, the moon has such a dramatic influence over life on Earth. The full scope of the moon's influence continues to evade scientific observation and dominate the human imagination and folklore the world over. The first example that comes immediately to mind is the ebb and flow of the tides, but the moon's magnetic pull applies equally well to all liquids on the planet, not just the sea. Arguably, that also includes the blood within our veins and the water within the cells of our physical bodies. Every wise farmer knows that the phases of the moon are of paramount importance in planting certain crops. Just look at any farmers' almanac, and you'll still see references to what phase the moon ought to be in when planting or harvesting certain crops. From the now classic book titled *Ozark Magic and Folklore* by author Vance Randolph, we see that "the changes of the moon and the signs of the zodiac are very important in determining the best dates for planting certain crops."[124] Randolph goes on to tell us that every mountain farmer knows that root vegetables do best when they are planted during the waning phase of the moon. Meanwhile, he also tells us that crops that bear their edible parts above ground tend to thrive better when they are planted during the waxing moon.[125]

Tarostar, an elder within the Sacred Pentagraph Tradition of Wicca and an occult author with nearly forty years' experience writing books about witchcraft, says, "The Moon is a signpost which indicates the prevailing direction of the life force, the reproductive energy that animates all living things … The Moon's vitality is either boosted, thwarted or channeled into specific areas of life, or away from them—all depending on Her position in the heavens."[126] As the moon waxes and wanes along its cosmic course, it unlocks access to subtle forces that the witch can channel and amplify within Circle.

---

124. Vance Randolph, *Ozark Magic and Folklore* (New York: Dover Publications, 1964), 34.

125. Randolph, *Ozark Magic and Folklore*, 34.

126. Tarostar, *The Sacred Pentagraph: Books IV & V*, 11.

- New moon—the perfect time to initiate a process, project, or start something new.

- Waxing moon—activate, empower, and work for any form of increase.

- Full moon—helps us bring things to a head or impede an action. This may seem odd to you at first, but when you consider that the moment something peaks, the only place for it to go from there is down, it is easier to see the influence that the full moon actually has upon our lives.

- Waning moon—brings a period of decrease and outright banishing before restarting the cycle again with the new moon.

By understanding the subtle mechanics associated with the moon's cycle, witches can harness greater power for their spells and rituals. When witches put themselves within the current of the present moment, they avoid fighting against the tide when seeking to accomplish their desires. Instead, they get the benefit of the natural energies present in the world around them at the time, augmenting their spells and rituals.

The Circle

The Circle is so vitally important to witchcraft. It has been called a temple, a container, a boundary, and so much more. Its value goes well beyond just being a simple temple for conducting sacred rites, though it certainly fills that function as well. Sometimes it does serve as a container to hold the energy raised within the circle. However, at other times, it acts more like a vortex, pulling ambient energy into its boundaries so that the witch can imprint his, her, or their will upon that energy, programming it with a specific intention. When it serves as a boundary, it demarcates the limits of a witch's microcosmic domain.

Like the athame, boline, cauldron, or broom, the Circle is actually one of the great tools of witchcraft. It assists witches in aligning the macrocosmic whole with their individual willpower. In Book IV of *The Sacred Pentagraph*, Tarostar says, "When a person sets out to strongly impress the Ether with his/her intense desire and firmly held visualizations he/she becomes a minor Creator/Creatrix of life."[127] While magic can certainly happen at any time, the formal process of casting the Circle helps focus the witch's thoughts and align the working with the intended purpose of the rite.

To make this witch's tool even more effective, an understanding of how energy moves is helpful. Think about the flow of energy in the universe like a cosmic river. Generally, this river flows positively, so the addition of a negative current will disrupt that flow briefly, rippling outward through the rest of the river until the natural order reestablishes itself. An effective Circle Cast does just that. It metaphorically disrupts the cosmic river's flow for a brief period so that the witch's will can ripple outward into the rest of creation.

Why Widdershins

Most traditions of witchcraft tend to cast their Circles deosil or clockwise today. I do not. Rather, I follow the teachings that were passed down to me during my initiations and cast my Circles widdershins or counterclockwise most of the time. There are only two times when I will cast the Circle deosil: during acts of protection and, as an extension of that, during exorcisms. Every other time, the Circle is cast widdershins.

Remember that the positive or electric current banishes what is already there. This topic was touched upon in chapter 4 in reference to the elements. However, because it seems to be such a unique way of looking at the witch's Circle for most of the witches I run into, it bears some further discussion before moving on to the events of an Esbat rite.

In order for witches to avoid draining their own vitality when powering their spells and workings, the ambient etheric power available in nature must be drawn into the Circle and then imbued with the witch's intention. This is where the widdershins or negative motion for casting the Circle comes into play. The negative motion of the widdershins Circle Cast draws the surrounding energy of the space into the witch's Circle, like a whirlpool or a vortex. By introducing an opposing current into the cosmic river of energy, which was discussed in this chapter's previous section, witches create a powerful vortex that provides them with more energy than their physical bodies alone could produce.

---

127. Tarostar, *The Sacred Pentagraph: Books IV & V*, 15.

When casting the Circle widdershins, begin in the north and move west, continuing one full circumambulation until arriving back in the north again. This is even more valuable if you ascribe the elements in the Circle-Cross format as discussed in chapter 4. However, on those rare occasions when the Circle is cast deosil, the witch begins in the east and moves toward the south, continuing one full circumambulation until arriving back in the east again.

When releasing the Circle back into the ether, the opposite motion is employed. Circles that were cast widdershins are released deosil, beginning in the east and circumambulating clockwise through the south back to the starting position in the east again. Circles that were cast deosil are released widdershins, beginning in the north and circumambulating counterclockwise through the west back to the starting position of the north again.

Through this method, the witch does a few very important things. First and foremost, if the Circle was cast widdershins, the positive action of releasing it deosil propels the energy out through the etheric or subtle realms to work the magick. A secondary benefit is that releasing the circle deosil also clears away or banishes any remaining effects of the witch's working after the energy has been sent off, returning the space back to its natural state. However, if the Circle was cast deosil to banish whatever baneful energy was present, the negative action of releasing the Circle widdershins after the protection or exorcism has been worked draws the natural energies back in to reclaim the space once again.

The Quarters

Again, the Circle-Cross format has the earth element in the north quarter, the water element in the west quarter, the fire element in the south quarter, and the air element in the east quarter. Since this format has been explained in depth in chapter 4, it's not necessary to elaborate upon it further here. What does need to be addressed now is that this format is not necessary to the proper casting of a witch's Circle. There are many branches of witchcraft that put the elements in other quarters.

One of my personal favorite variations involves placing the elements according to the witch's immediate orientation in the world at that moment of the ritual. It feels so very hedge witch to me, like I'm working directly with my land spirits each time I do it. For example, I live on the East Coast of the United States. Therefore, because the Atlantic Ocean is to the east of me, water would take up the east quarter in my Circles. The equator, or the hottest point on the globe in relation to my location, would take up my south quarter. The great expanse of the continent and the Rocky Mountains lie west of me, so the earth element would take up my west quarter, and, since air exists all around us, the air element would take up the last remaining quarter in the north of my Circle.

Some branches of witchcraft don't ascribe any elements to the quarters at all. Instead, the witches who subscribe to this philosophy operate by merely demarcating their boundary and getting immediately to the task at hand. The elegance of that approach really does have to be appreciated.

While I appreciate and even love the other approaches, I have to admit that I still favor the Circle-Cross format, because of its metaphysical implications. The idea of reproducing the act of creation through the positive expansive motion and undoing creation to take us back to the Void or Deity through the negative magnetic motion is endlessly fascinating to me. The eternal dance between the two cosmic forces in each ritual feels so primal, so powerful to me. It sparks my creative imagination in a way that none of the other methods manage to do. In this case, pick the version that works best for you. As long as you understand the metaphysical mechanics behind the Circle Cast and you adhere to some basic principles, the trappings of the Circle can be played around with a little bit.

Elementals & the Witch's Circle

In addition to delineating a boundary for the witch's microcosm, a good solid Circle Cast, and the ritual that follows it, will stir the astral light. That is, these actions will call forth the elementals from the astral realm, and, once the elementals have arrived, they will work with the witch to accomplish the desired intention for the spell or ritual.

The elementals are drawn to the trappings of ritual like moths to a flame. They love the incense, the bright colors, the earthly representations of the elements, and the various other correspondences that have become a part of witchcraft. In fact, it is because of the magnetic pull that these things have over the elementals that they have become part of witchcraft in the first place.

While witches tend to talk about the elementals as if they are sentient anthropomorphic beings, that's not, strictly speaking, true. Some elementals have grown beyond their natural state into something more. They did this by consistently working with people on a specific intention over a prolonged and extended period of time. However, in their natural state, elementals function more like power cells. I like to think of them as the stem cells of the astral plane. Just like stem cells in the physical body, the elementals are malleable and ready to be programmed to do a variety of specific functions or tasks. Some occult writers have chosen the term *elementaries* to refer to the elementals in their natural, preprogrammed state. These same writers have reserved the term *elemental* for more anthropomorphic beings. For the sake of clarity, that makes sense.

One of the reasons that elementaries are drawn to the trappings of ritual is because the trappings themselves are indicative of human thought and feeling. Each elementary has a program within itself, like DNA, to become more than its base potential. In its natural state, it is just undifferentiated energy, like a battery that is hooked up to provide power to something. That same battery can be used to power a flashlight or the clock that hangs on your wall. It doesn't matter to the battery how its storehouse of energy is used. This is an elementary in its natural state. However, each elementary "seeks" to have a life outside of this base existence, to become an elemental or more. To do that, it needs human thought.

This is the power of the witch. By working with witches and other magickal people, the elementary gets combined with a human thought and becomes an elemental, sometimes called a *thoughtform elemental*. The more powerful the thought and the more potent the emotion behind that thought, the more draw it has for the elementaries. More powerful thoughts and stronger emotions draw more potent elementaries—that is, more powerful thoughts draw a greater storehouse of power.

When the elementaries latch on to the human thought, the thoughtform that is created through this merging lasts as long as the storehouse of energy exists to power it. This is why some thoughts seem to pervade all of society and others are fleeting. For example, the thoughtform surrounding the concept of "Life, liberty, and the pursuit of happiness" or the fear that surrounded the Covid-19 crisis are/were both extremely powerful thoughtforms. That is, these thoughts are/were pulled from a large storehouse of energy provided by very powerful elementaries. Meanwhile, other thoughts, like the thought about what you might have for breakfast, are rather weak thoughts and don't draw the elementaries as readily. Therefore, they are fleeting, because once the little bit of elementary energy they do manage to draw wears out, people simply forget the idea completely.

As time goes on, some of these more powerful thoughtforms last long enough and become influential enough over a large enough group of people that they get concretized in myth and legend. When this happens, they succeed at evolving into independent elemental beings, like the various fairylike beings who regularly work with witches.

Many witches ask why these great beings would even deign to work with humans in the first place. This is why. Without human thought and the emotional energy that recharges the elementary batteries of these beings, they lose their power and begin to disappear back into the astral light. By working with witches, the elemental beings exceed their original programming. By maintaining a relationship with witches, these elemental beings constantly repower their elementary cells.

The Circle-Cross format seems extremely effective at drawing the elemental energies, which is yet another reason why I love it so much. However, any ritual that you put a great deal of thought into will work according to the power of the thought you put in. This is what some witches mean when they talk about intention. That is to say, if witches solidify their wills around a desired outcome, they choose the appropriate correspondences for that specified desire, they add the appropriate ritual gestures and other trappings in line with the specified desire, and so on, they will succeed at drawing these powerful elementary batteries to their Circles.

The Horned God & the Goddess

I don't generally invoke both the Horned God and Goddess at each Esbat, because I believe that the gods are personified principles, representative of two primal energies of creation—fire and ice, positive and negative, electric and magnetic, and so on. These energies balance each other out and, together, create the objective realms of existence. Because of that belief, I tend to channel one or the other Principle Energy as the case requires.

At the new and waning phases of the moon's concourse, I work with the Horned God and his energies. During the waning period from full back to new, I work with the Goddess and her energies. In this way, I better narrow the focus of my intention for each spell, the relationship between me and the Horned God during an Esbat being yet another correspondence to communicate my desire to initiate something or work for positive increase. Conversely, my interaction with the Goddess during the full and waning moon Esbats signals my opposite intention to the subtle realms.

The Godforce, whatever name you give him, initiates cycles, brings order out of chaos, and so on. In Hermetic terms, he is connected to the positive, electric, and expansive energies of the universe. In Theosophical terms, it was the God that brought movement to the Void and initiated the process of creation.[128] We see this same theme repeated in the story of Lucifer and Diana from Charles G. Leland's classic *Aradia or Gospel of the Witches*.[129] After the separation occurred, it was Lucifer's explosive escape out of the Void that brought about creation. Science calls this *the big bang*. Meanwhile the Goddess and her energetic current are seen as the opposite. In Hermetic terms, she is connected to the negative, magnetic, and constrictive current, taking us back into the Void, back into the unification of the All. In Theosophical terms, it is the Goddess who returns the objective universe back to the subjective, taking everything back to the All once more.[130]

There is a paradox here that is worth further study. While the Goddess grants life, she is also the force that takes that life away again. She slows down matter, condensing it into material form and banishing the physical realm back into the Void, returning us to a unified whole once more.

Like the branch of witchcraft I was initiated into, the deities are viewed as principles within yoga practice and theory. These Divine Principles can be worked with to bring out corresponding currents within the yogi. A similar phenomenon occurs within the witch's magickal practice when the gods are approached in this way.

I have added two sets of yoga practices to this chapter to help witches do just that. It is not essential that witches subscribe to my view of witchcraft to get the benefit of these practices. They will work equally well for the die-hard polytheistic witch as they do for the witch who buys into the idea that the gods are principles—personified or otherwise.

---

128. Blavatsky, *The Key to Theosophy*, 50.

129. Leadbetter, *Aradia*, 41–44.

130. Blavatsky, *The Key to Theosophy*, 50.

The first sequence is designed to be done anytime during the new and waxing moons in order to better connect with the Godforce or the electric current. The second sequence is designed to be done anytime during the full and waning moons in order to better connect with the Goddess energies or the magnetic current. Both sequences may be done before the ritual or they may be used in place of a verbal invocation to the specific god or goddess being worked with during the ritual.

The New & Waxing Moons

The new moon is dedicated to the Horned God, because it is positive in nature. During the new moon, the sun and moon are conjunct, so their power is aligned. They share in each other's essence. Some witches refer to this phase as *The Dark of the Moon* or simply *The Dark Moon*. Regardless of what it is called, its energy mirrors the positive, expansive force that initiated creation. This was discussed earlier in regard to the elements in chapter 4 as well. Like the explosive energy of creation, the new moon initiates a period of increase that expands the lunar light and the positive current available for witches to use through the waxing phase into the moon's fullness. It is the primary time for enchantments and spells for anything beneficial in nature.[131] This is a wonderful time to work for increase or growth in all areas of life. It's also the Esbat associated with the largest variety of spells.

The God Sequence

This sequence is really more of a pose than a sequence. It may be done whenever a witch desires to align with the Horned God's energy or has need of the positive, electric energetic current of creation. Better that this yoga pose be performed during the period between the new and waxing moons, since it will align the witch's energy with the natural cycles available at the time.

Simhasana, which translates as *lion pose* or *lion's breath pose*, is so common place that most people who have been taking yoga for more than a month or two have probably seen this pose. It's relatively easy, but in the beginning some people may feel self-conscious or insecure, because it can seem a bit silly to Western minds that are

---

131. Tarostar, *Sacred Pentagraph: Books IV & V*, 13.

used to being very in control and always conditioned to look good. However, because of this pose's ability to invigorate the body, increase vitality, and project the mind outward, it is absolutely perfect for connecting with the Horned God, Godforce, or the electric current.

On the day of the new or waxing moon Esbat, perform this exercise facing the sun, absorbing some of the etheric energy coming from the sun's rays. It would be best to perform the exercise outside. Though only one round of this exercise needs to be done for success, the effect is cumulative when done several times throughout the day. Start slow; only do the exercise once or twice before a ritual, but as your meditation skills grow and your imaginative will strengthens, add more rounds. Some witches perform this exercise every hour between sunrise and sunset on the day of their Esbat rite.

Imagine yourself to be surrounded by a fiery sphere or orb. With your active imagination, tell yourself that the fiery sphere is the primal electric energy of creation all around you. As you begin to inhale, breathe in the fire element. Inhale through the nose and through every pore on your skin. Imagine the fire energy circulating around your body before you exhale. As you exhale, empty your mind of all thoughts.

1. Sit in a simple, cross-legged position (also called *padmasana* or *lotus pose*) on the floor and place your palms down on the ground in front of your shins. Spread the fingers wide and press the palms into the ground. Keep all parts of your palm in contact with the floor. Do not curl your fingers. Straighten the arms and arch your back slightly. This is a subtle movement. If you find that you are pushing your belly out in front of you, you are arching too much. You want your back in a neutral position, nearly straight but without the normal stress or strain that comes along with holding your back rigid. Tilt the pelvis slightly forward so that you are leaning into your hands, and lift your chest up toward the sky. Finally, lift your chin slightly and, with your eyes open, look upward at your third eye. All of this together is the starting position.

2. With your mouth closed, curl your tongue upward so that the tip and a bit of the underside of the tongue press firmly against the palate. Maintain the pressure during the long, slow, deep inhalation through the nose.

3. On the exhale, open your mouth suddenly and quickly push the tongue out of the mouth as far as you can. At the same time, verbalize the seed syllable *aaahhhh* in a breathy tone. Close the mouth.

4. Inhale again, and continue the process for three to seven repetitions before uncrossing your legs and repeating the entire exercise with the other leg crossed in front. Both sides balanced out in this way constitutes one round of this exercise.

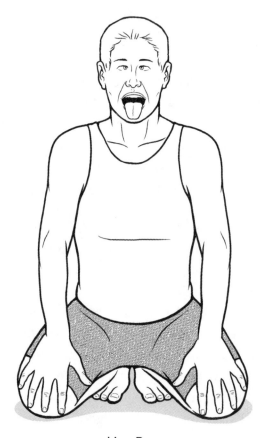

Lion Pose

Another alternative visualization for witches who struggle with fire imagery is to visualize yourself as the Horned God. Feel yourself growing hotter, taking on the primal heat and expansive quality of the electric current. Maybe you even feel yourself growing bigger and expanding outward further and further beyond the limits of the physical body with each exhalation. For male witches, you may feel yourself become physically aroused. For female, transgender, or gender-fluid witches, it might be useful to ask yourself how you connect with your internal masculine.

The Full & Waning Moons

The full moon is the point in the lunar course where the energy peaks and things are brought to fruition. It's an excellent time for manifestation or concluding any situation. The energies associated with these phases are also good for banishing, deflating, or impeding.[132] The Goddess energy serves as both Creatrix and Destroyer, and the energies of the full and waning moons partake of her essence. As the full moon peaks, projects are brought to their conclusion and the successful outcome of a goal can be reached. As the waning moon decreases, obstacles can be removed from a witch's path. In this way, the full and waning moons partake of the Goddess's role as Mother or Creatrix of Life and Destroyer.

The Goddess Sequence

Hatha yoga is the prevailing style of yoga in the West. It is the one that most of us are familiar with, but it is not the only style available to help witches develop along their magickal paths. The mind turns inward with a Hatha yoga practice. Turning inward and drawing attention into that still small point of focus within, concentrating on the vast nothingness of an empty mind is wonderful for charging ourselves magnetically. It makes us the center of our own microcosm, giving us our own etheric or spiritual version of gravitational pull, so to speak.

While the Horned God sequence was a bit more active, the Goddess sequence places your body in a passive position. Whereas the God sequence invoked the primal element of fire to produce heat and put you in sympathy with the electric current, the Goddess sequence is designed to invoke the primal element of water to produce a cooling effect and put the witch in sympathy with the magnetic current.

---

132. Tarostar, *Sacred Pentagraph: Books IV & V*, 14.

Though the body will be completely passive in one position for this entire exercise, the mind will turn inward in order to create a microcosmic world, magnetizing the body. In this way, the witch becomes more like the Goddess, operating in sympathy with her energies.

Anyone who has ever taken a yoga class in a gym or studio may be familiar with this pose. It's called *reclining bound angle pose* or *supta baddha konasana*. With the soles of the feet touching and pulled in close to the groin, this pose mimics giving birth and is a wonderful way to connect with the Goddess's energy.

1. About ten to fifteen minutes before you desire to go into ritual to do a full moon Esbat, lie down on the ground supine or faceup.

2. Bend your knees, keeping them together while the soles of your feet are pressed against the ground.

3. Touch the soles of your feet together, and allow your knees to fall gently to the ground, creating a geometric shape that looks roughly like a diamond with the empty space between the knees.

4. Close your eyes, and allow your mind to turn inward. Imagine yourself floating on a vast and infinite ocean, just like in chapter 8 for the exercise on developing clairsentience. See this ocean as a vast expanse of cold darkness.

5. After about ten minutes of quiet relaxation, focus on breathing in the coldness of the water element. Feel the coldness rushing into your body. Allow yourself to fill up with that cold, constricting energy. Feel yourself getting heavier, condensing. You may actually even feel your body tense up slightly, like when you enter a pool and the water is colder than expected. Really allow yourself to live this experience for a moment. Tell yourself that the cold and constricting feeling is symbolic of the magnetic pull of the cosmos. Do this for no more than seven deep belly breaths. During those seven breaths, magnetize every cell in the body, infusing it with Goddess energy. Maybe even see yourself taking on characteristics or qualities that align with your version of the Goddess.

6. Then perform your spell or ritual. After the ritual, return to this position; relax yourself again fully. Imagine that you are once again floating upon the vast and infinite ocean of cold darkness. Release the cold, constrictive energy back into the infinite expanse all around you. Feel your body beginning to warm up, returning to normal. Then partake of the witch's post-ritual feast in order to ground yourself.

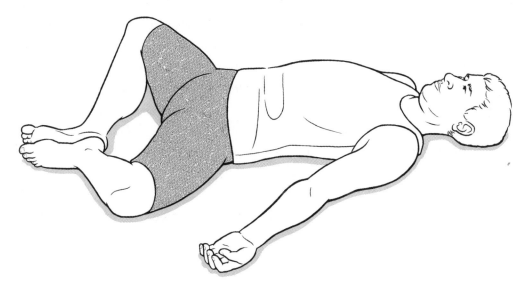

Reclining Bound Angle Pose

Don't feel confined by the visualization described here. The fear of water is very real, and for some people, that might be just enough to prevent them from tapping into this wonderful Goddess energy. If you are one of the witches who struggle with a fear of water, it might be useful to simply imagine yourself growing colder and colder, taking on the primal coldness of the magnetic current. Visualize yourself as the Goddess as you see her. For female witches, it might even be useful to see yourself giving birth. For male, transgender, and gender-fluid witches, it might be useful to ask yourself how you connect with your internal feminine.

Adding Yoga

These two sequences for getting in sympathy with the electric and magnetic currents of the Horned God and the Goddess are not the only ways to add yoga into your witchcraft practice. There are also pranayama or breathing techniques that can be added to your spell work. A few different pranayama-style exercises have been provided in this book, but this is a vast topic. It's actually one entire branch of yoga on its own, and whole volumes of books could be written on it. If you would like to explore the topic further, there are some wonderful resources in the Recommended Reading section at the back of this book that will help you begin that exploration. There are also other Hatha-style yoga poses and sequences that can be used before or during ritual to better align the witch with the ritual's intended purpose. Some of those sequences can be found in this book's last chapter, though, again, the possibilities for combining yoga and magick in this way are endless. For a cunning witch who understands the documented purpose of each pose or sequence of poses, there is no limit to the manner in which this aspect of yoga can benefit a magickal practice.

10

YOGA & THE WHEEL
OF THE YEAR

The witch's sabbatic cycle works sort of like a battery. By balancing the opposites of action and reaction through the Wheel of the Year, the witch continues to grow in power with each turn of the Wheel. I like to think of this process like charging a kinetic watch. By regular and consistent movement through the Wheel, the witch's personal batteries are constantly recharged and sustained.

As I was taught in the coven into which I was initiated, the four solar sabbats are symbolic of birth, life, death, and regeneration. These sabbats share in God's power and tell his story, which mirrors our own mysterious journey through reincarnation and spiritual evolution toward an eventual enlightenment. Those sabbats coincide with the solstices and equinoxes. Just as God is the Divine Initiator who unlocks the creative process, the solar sabbats initiate a change in the cosmos, which the earth responds to. As the light increases upon the land, life flourishes and an eventual bountiful harvest is reaped. The four terrestrial sabbats or cross-quarter days play off the themes of fertility and abundance. Thus, they belong to the Goddess. Hallowmas, Candlemas or Imbolc, Beltane, and Lammas are her rites. The coven where I was initiated used (and still uses) Tarostar's *Sacred Pentagraph Books* a great deal, and all of this information can be found in much greater detail within those books, but for the purposes of this book on yoga and witchcraft, this brief overview of seasonal interactions should suffice.[133]

As time goes on, the witch who keeps the sabbats in this way grows in psychic power. Eventually this power can increase to such an extent that physical world manifestations can sometimes occur. I have personally seen adept witches move dowsing rods with nothing but the power of their minds. I know of at least two witches who were able to make a flame jump from one taper to another without the two candles touching. The witch whom I saw exercise this power was able to light the second candle from nearly a foot away. Personally, I have even astral projected great distances to check up on people I love. Later on, those same people call me with "the most interesting story" or asking if I was in their area on the day in question. No amount of convincing them that I wasn't ever does the trick. I even know of cases where entire covens are able to share the same dream and recount the details exactly to each other in the waking world. The addition of yoga to the witch's Wheel of the Year can greatly accelerate the growth of these psychic powers.

While there aren't specific yoga poses that necessarily pair with each season, this fact does not have to present an obstacle to witches who wish to pair a yoga practice with their Wheel of the Year celebrations. Yoga teacher training programs spend a great deal of time teaching yoga instructors how to theme a class, because the best yoga classes are built off themes. Truthfully, theming a class has always been one of my favorite aspects of teaching yoga, and there are more than enough themes happening in the mythologies surrounding the witch's Wheel of the Year for witches to work with. As time goes by, it may be appropriate for some witches who want to deepen their practice to take a workshop or class on theming a yoga class. Once the basic skill is learned, the possibilities for nurturing the basic seed thought of adding yoga sequences to witchcraft can be cultivated further.

---

133. Tarostar, *Sacred Pentagraph: Books I, II & III*, 149.

Yoga & the Witch's Sabbats

There are several possible starting points on the traditional Wheel of the Year. Some witches start with Samhain, which they view as the witch's New Year. My tradition has always called that rite *Hallowmas*, and that is how I prefer to think of it, but if you are drawn to a more Celtic style of witchcraft, it is completely appropriate to refer to this ritual as *Samhain*. Some witches start the Wheel of the Year at the darkest point in the year: Yule or the winter solstice. When this point is chosen as the starting point, the theory is that all life starts in darkness. The baby in the mother's womb and the seed planted in the ground—both require an initial period of darkness to thrive when they finally emerge into the light. Another common place to begin the Wheel of the Year is at Imbolc or, as my tradition refers to this sabbat, Candlemas. The theory behind this position as the starting point is that it's easier to recognize new life at the moment of birth or when plants begin to flower.

I have chosen Hallowmas as the starting point for this version of the Wheel for two reasons. First, it's what most witches have come to expect in public material on witchcraft, and second, I love the symbolism that comes with starting over at a point of regeneration. It just feels so uplifting, but for witches who are already part of a tradition or who already have established their own magickal practice, honor that. Start where it has become tradition to start. Ultimately, the beauty of the Wheel is that there is no beginning or ending.

Hallowmas

Hallowmas, also called *Samhain* or *The Witch's New Year* in some traditions, actually ends the cycles of both the solar and the terrestrial sabbats. However, many witches tend to think of it as the beginning of the Wheel of the Year, which is okay. The end of one cycle is the beginning of another. That's just how the law of rhythm works.[134]

Hallowmas is symbolic of the Void. It is the primal darkness before the light was created, and, as such, it takes death as its primary theme. The Wild Hunt, the Day of the Dead, or working with the fair folk—this season is intimately connected with the Veil between this world and the next and all that is associated with it.

---

134. Deslippe, *The Kybalion*, 269–83.

A Yoga Sequence for Hallowmas

In order to communicate with the dead, whether they be astral shades, ancestors, or spirits, witches must develop their psychic powers. This sequence only has one meditative pose, but it only needs the one. On a psychic level, it turbocharges the work done earlier in this book and prepares witches for their upcoming Hallowmas ritual.

Because of its peaceful, contemplative nature, it would be appropriate to perform this meditation roughly ten to twenty minutes before the beginning of your Hallowmas ritual. This simple meditation combines a mudra and a chant designed to connect you with your Higher Self and clear your consciousness so that you can become aware of the psychic messages you are receiving.

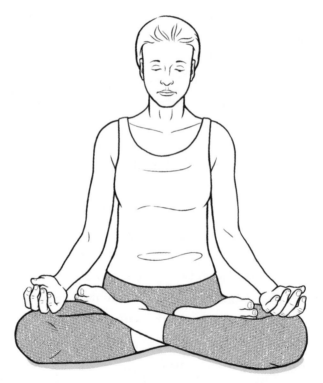

Lotus Pose

1. When you are ready to begin your meditation for psychic development, sit with a straight back, allowing your shoulders to "float" easily over the hips in a cross-

legged position (lotus pose). Eliminate all tension in your back. Alternatively, you may choose to sit with your back against a wall. Place your hands gently on your thighs with your palms facing up. Touch the tips of your pointer finger to the thumb on each hand, and allow the other three fingers to extend out naturally. This is called *om mudra* or *chin mudra*.

2. Chant the sacred *OM* (pronounced *oh-mmmmmmm*) by taking a deep belly breath in through the nose and vocalizing the sacred sound as you exhale. Continue this practice for as long as you can during your meditation. Take breathing breaks whenever you need them.

The Winter Solstice

The winter solstice, also known as Yule, is a solar rite where the light begins its journey back out of darkness. It is a time of hope and anticipation for the possibilities that are yet to come. This is actually a period of stasis and reflection. It's a time to clear away that which no longer serves and to make way for new possibilities that can manifest with the increasing light.

A Yoga Sequence for the Winter Solstice

Unlike the Hallowmas meditation, this sequence gets you up and moving and brings you back to life. In a sense, it mirrors the rebirth of the sun on a personal level. Ideally, you would wake up and greet the dawn as you do this series of poses. *Surya namaskar A*, also called *sun salutation A*, is a series of poses that is designed to create a flow of movement within the body. Each pose is coordinated with the breath. You inhale into one pose and exhale into the next as you flow through all ten postures. Like the sun that brings light and life back to the earth, these poses invigorate us while building heat within the body.

1. Stand in mountain pose (tadasana) with your feet firmly pressed against the earth, your knees close together, and your hands in prayer position at the heart chakra.

2. Inhale as you sweep your arms out to your side and bring them up above your head in a gentle flowing arch. As your hands come together, gently lift your chest, arching your back, and look up at your thumbs.

3. Exhale as you fold forward (uttanasana), hinging at the hips in a swan dive motion. Bring your nose as close to your knees as your body will let you. Allow your hands to hang loose and limp by your ankles.

4. On your next inhale, lift your chest away from your thighs and keep the back straight, lengthening your spine by pressing the crown of your head toward the front of the mat. Elongate the neck and the spine, flattening out your back as you come into a standing half forward bend (ardha uttanasana). Imagine that your back is like a table with two legs. You want to create a surface flat enough to eat off of.

5. Exhale as you place your hands on the mat and step or jump back into plank pose. Place your hands directly under your shoulders and your feet hip distance apart. Continue exhaling as you lower your body down to the ground in one smooth, fluid motion, moving to the rhythm of your exhalation. The full motion involved in this pose is called *chaturanga*.

6. As you inhale, pull your chest up as you press your hands into the mat and straighten your arms. You should have a slight curve in your lower back as you press the tops of your feet into the mat and lift your thighs up off the mat into upward-facing dog (urdhva mukha svanasana).

7. As you exhale, lift your hips and roll back over your toes, placing the soles of your feet firmly on the ground as you press your sit bones back toward the rear end of your mat. While doing that, straighten your arms and firmly press your palms into the mat, pushing your weight back onto your feet as you lengthen your spine. Your heels do not have to touch down, and you can certainly bend your knees slightly if you need to. Take a moment here in downward-facing dog pose (adho mukha svanasana) and look at a spot on the mat between your hands before moving on. Even if that means you need to take another full breath before flowing to the next posture, that's okay.

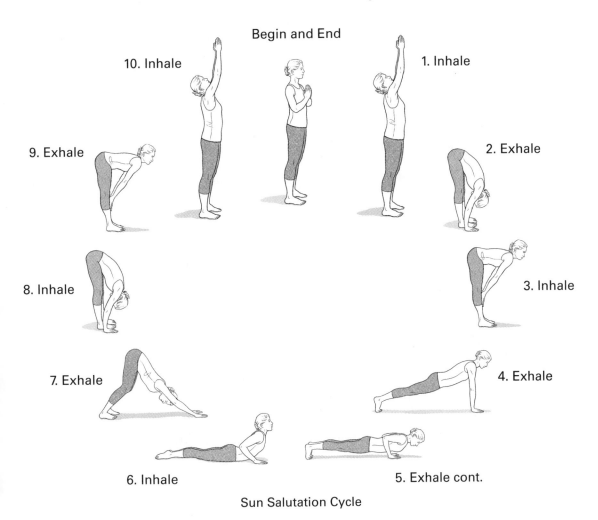

Begin and End

10. Inhale

1. Inhale

9. Exhale

2. Exhale

8. Inhale

3. Inhale

7. Exhale

4. Exhale

6. Inhale

5. Exhale cont.

Sun Salutation Cycle

8. Inhale as you step or jump forward, placing both feet between your hands at the front of your mat. Lift your torso halfway up, and as you do so, lengthen your spine, pushing your sit bones toward the back of the mat as you elongate your neck and press the crown of your head toward the front of the mat. This should flatten your back. Ideally, you would keep your hands on the floor, but it is also acceptable to place them on your shins. What matters more is that your back stays flat in this position.

9. Exhale into a standing forward fold (uttanasana) again. Bring your nose close to your knees as you let your hands hang loose and limp by your ankles.

10. Inhale as you reverse your swan dive, sweeping your arms out to the side as you reverse the hinge of the hips, extending up to a standing position once again. Continue sweeping your hands up above your head until the palms touch, and give a slight back bend as you gaze up at your thumbs.

11. Exhale your hands back to prayer position and find yourself back in tadasana where you started.

Candlemas

While many witches celebrate Imbolc during this time of the year, the tradition where I learned witchcraft does not. Imbolc is a specific holiday tied to a Celtic mythology and the goddess Brigid. However, since this season is relevant to all witches, not just Celtic witches, I prefer to use the more universal term for this season, which is why I tend to celebrate Candlemas instead.

This sabbat responds to the midwinter rite. In reproductive terms, this is when the womb is prepared to conceive, and mother's milk begins to flow. However, it is so much more than that. On a purely metaphysical level, this is the moment when conditions are ripe for manifestation. This is when the energetic possibilities of midwinter become manifest into matter. The first flowers of spring even begin to appear across the landscape in some climates.

A Yoga Sequence for Candlemas

Below you will find a wonderful sequence of poses for manifestation. Before we can manifest anything, we must first know that which we desire to see brought into existence. On the most basic surface level, this process talks about reproduction and concretizing energy into the physical form of a baby or offspring. However, that is not the full scope of this process. It also includes the creation of "thought babies"—great works of art, literature, science, and so much more. Our civilization and our species are advanced through all these creative acts, just as they are by rearing up the next generation.

Roughly about two weeks before your Imbolc ritual, begin this yoga sequence for manifesting your desires. If you do not already know what you wish to manifest or create, use your contemplative time at the beginning of this sequence to focus your mind on these topics, and allow something to come to you intuitively over the course of the two weeks prior to the ritual. If you already know your heart's desire going into this two-week period, spend your time at the beginning of this sequence concentrating intensely upon that desire. Imagine it already in your life. See yourself interacting with it. See your life better because you've successfully achieved that which you set your mind upon now. This brings up a good point. You should be holding your intention firmly in your mind as you move through all the poses in this sequence of poses. (The same is true for the sequences connected with the other sabbats.) Perform this sequence roughly twenty to thirty minutes before your ritual on the final night.

1. Begin in easy pose (sukhasana) with your legs crossed in front of you on the floor. Lengthen your spine and keep your back straight as you stack your shoulders above your hips. Place your hands (one on top of the other) in your lap with your palms facing upward, and contemplate your intention for your upcoming Imbolc rite.

2. When you have meditated on your intention and you have lost your concentration (somewhere between five and ten minutes), come up into a simple tabletop position with your hands under your shoulders and your thighs hip distance apart with your knees directly under your hip bones. Bring the big toes of both feet together and, as you exhale, allow your torso to sink between your thighs. Flatten your lower back as you push your tailbone toward the back of the mat and press the crown of your head forward, allowing your forehead to come to a resting position on the mat. Lay your arms on the mat by your legs with your palms up, and allow your shoulders to roll gently forward so that you round the upper part of your back, and find yourself resting in child's pose (balasana). Alternatively, you can reach your arms out for the front of the mat and flatten your torso against the ground. Do what feels right for your body.

3. On an inhale, come back up into a tabletop position, bringing your chest forward between your hands and lowering your body back down to the mat with your chest pressed against the floor on the exhalation. Stretch your legs back, and press the tops of your feet into the mat or ground beneath you. Reposition your hands so that they are under your shoulders and squeeze your elbows in close to your sides. Firmly press the feet, the thighs, and the pelvis into the mat. As you inhale, straighten your arms, press your hands firmly into the mat, and lift your torso off the mat, but keep your lower body (starting at least at your pelvis) in contact with the earth. Finally, roll your shoulders down away from your ears as you squeeze your shoulder blades and lift your chest to the sky. This is cobra pose (bhujangasana). Take five to ten deep belly breaths here before lowering your chest back down to the mat beneath you on an exhalation.

4. Find yourself again with your belly and chest flat against the mat beneath you, your arms by your sides with your palms facing up toward the sky (your thumbs should be grazing your thighs). Traditional versions of this pose ask for your forehead to be pressed against the ground, but some people find that uncomfortable. If you find that you have to turn your head for your own comfort in the prone position, just make sure to balance out each side so that you don't strain your neck. Rotate your thighs by simply turning your big toes toward each other, and squeeze your glutes together. This is the beginning of locust pose (salabhasana). On an exhale, lift your head, shoulders, and legs below the knee, and forearms up off the mat. Press your lower abdomen, pelvis, and thighs into the ground. Stay in this active portion of the pose for thirty seconds to a minute before releasing back down to the starting position on an exhale. Repeat two or three more times before moving on to the next pose.

5. On an inhale, come back up to a tabletop position and follow the instructions above for moving back into child's pose (balasana).

Child's pose is an excellent way to finish a yoga sequence. It releases tension in the back, which so many people suffer with in the modern world. It releases stress and anxiety, and it produces a general sense of physical, mental, and emotional relief. This is one of the nicest resting poses a witch can do before ritual, because it allows you to completely relax without having to lie down flat on the ground.

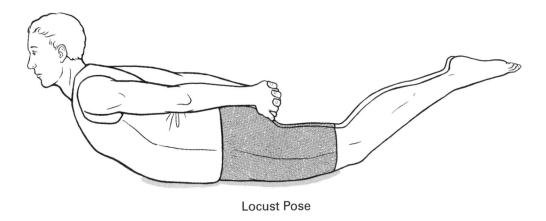

Locust Pose

The Spring Equinox

This sabbat is masculine or projective in nature. It celebrates the joy of youth and the abundance of budding life. It's a time for new beginnings and planting the seeds of things you wish to see manifest in your life.

A Yoga Sequence for the Spring Equinox

The energies of spring surge forth. Animals feel it. Plants pollinate in order to spread their seed. Even people get a little more randy as the light comes back and the weather warms up. This sequence of yoga poses is designed to help you increase your libido and raise some of that powerful energy out of your root chakra so that you can use it to power your new projects. The best time to do this practice is in the early morning right when you wake up so that you can enjoy the benefits of vitality that it brings.

1. Start in tabletop on your hands and knees with your hands directly under your shoulders and your knees directly under your hips about hip distance apart. Now, focusing on the root chakra, concentrate on squeezing the muscles of the pelvic floor, like you are trying to stop the flow of urine. Hold for five

seconds and then release. Repeat this process roughly ten times as you concentrate on your spring rite intention.

2. As you inhale, arch your back and drop the belly so that you look like a cow with its udders hanging down close to the ground. As you exhale, pull the belly button in close to the spine, rounding your back and pushing your shoulder blades up toward the sky so that you look like a cat. Move through these two postures in line with your breath.

3. Curl your toes under (if they are not already in that position) and press your palms firmly into the mat. Lift your hips up to the sky as you straighten the legs and press your sit bones back, lengthening the spine and creating an upside-down *V* with your body. Take ten to twenty deep belly breaths here.

4. Come back down to your hands and knees and then make your way onto your back. Allow yourself to rest with your back against the mat or ground for a few more moments. Let go of all control of your breath, and just focus on the intention for your upcoming rite. Feel your body surging with the primal energy of your root chakra.

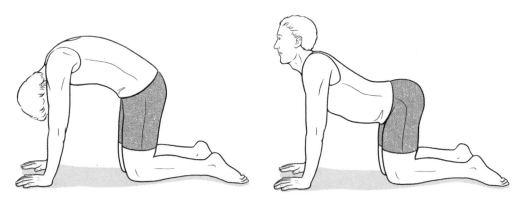

Cat-Cow Pose

Beltane

As a response to the abundant joy of the spring equinox, Beltane is seen as the glory of life in full bloom, represented by the maiden goddesses. What started out as a young infatuation or flirtation has blossomed into something truly beautiful. Good luck and blessings abound during this season.

A Yoga Sequence for Beltane

Beltane is all about the beauty of life, and who doesn't want to be more radiantly beautiful! Witches of old used to wake up at dawn on the first day of May and wash their faces in the early morning dew. If you live in an environment that allows you to practice yoga outside on the grass that early in the morning, it might be a wonderful idea to take your Beltane yoga sequence outside and take advantage of this wonderful custom for youthful beauty.

We are all beautiful in our own way, but our insecurities often make us discount that unique beauty. This yoga sequence and the visualizations that go with it will help you take control of the things that you see as "imperfections" and transmute them into beauty you can appreciate. Be kind to yourself.

1. Start by lying facedown on the ground. You can use a yoga mat if you prefer so that you don't slip and slide on the grass, but make sure that your head is off the mat. (Some people find yoga mats to be more problematic than they're worth when practicing outside. Whether you use a mat or not is entirely up to you. Personally, I don't generally use them outside when practicing on the grass.) That way the dew from the grass can moisten your face. Imagine that the dew is rejuvenating you. As you breathe in and out, visualize yourself growing more and more beautiful with each inhalation. See yourself the way you want to look, use your imaginative will to correct any minor imperfections or blemishes. As you imagine yourself getting more and more beautiful than you already are, repeat an affirmation to yourself that reaffirms this fact to your subconscious mind. As you exhale, empty your mind of all thoughts

and just feel the movement of your breath. Repeat for as long as you need to in order to feel the magick of the May Day dew rejuvenating you.

2. When you are ready to move on with your practice, bring your hands underneath your shoulders and curl your toes under so that you can press yourself up into a plank position. Lift your hips to the sky and press your sit bones back as far as you can. Your heels do not have to touch the mat. It is also appropriate to bend your knees slightly, if the tension in the back of your legs becomes too intense. While pushing back, straighten your arms and firmly press your palms into the mat. This will readjust your weight back onto your feet. Lengthen your spine as you pull your shoulders down away from your ears. When you have fully gotten into the pose, allow your mind to turn inward. Take a moment here in downward-facing dog pose (adho mukha svanasana) to concentrate on your own beauty as you allow the blood to flow into the face, which will help you look your best. See the same image you just saw when you moistened your face with the morning dew in step 1.

3. On an inhale, step, walk, or jump your feet between your hands. Lift your torso halfway up, and as you do so, lengthen your spine. You want to create a flat surface with your back, like a tabletop. Place your hands on your shins or thighs and press your sit bones back away from your shoulders. Really elongate your spine as much as possible. This includes your neck. Try to pull your ears forward and away from your shoulders by pressing the crown of your head as far in front of you as possible. You should feel a sense of dynamic tension in your torso and a slight stretch along the backs of the legs.

4. Exhale into a standing forward fold (uttanasana). Bring your nose as close to your knees as you are able to. Let your hands hang loose and limp by your ankles. Alternatively, you can wrap your arms around your legs and give yourself a hug. Stay in this pose as long as it is comfortable for you. As an inversion where your head is below your hips, this pose infuses the facial tissues with blood, plumping them up and making you more beautiful.

5. On an inhale, slowly roll yourself up into a standing position. Take this very slowly. In your mind, you may want to count from one to ten as you rise up.

Take the full ten seconds. Don't rush the process. Start by just tucking the tailbone. Then pull your belly button in close to your spine to support your rising action. Allow your upper body to uncurl naturally. Roll the shoulders back and down as you pull the shoulder blades in close against your spine. Untuck your chin from your chest so that it is parallel to the ground.

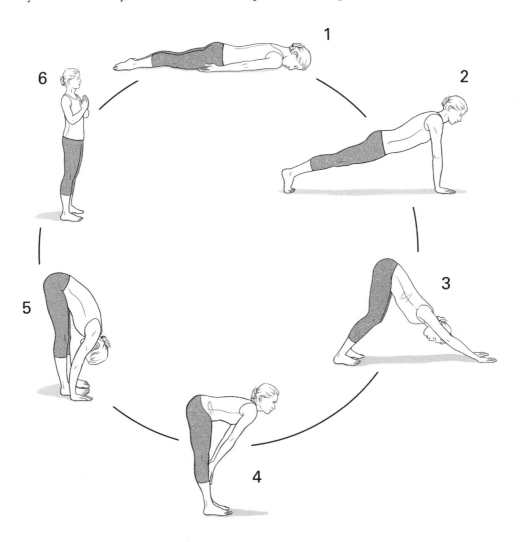

Beltane Sequence

It is extremely important that you take the process of coming up out of a standing forward fold very slowly. This is especially true if you have any medical conditions that might be exacerbated by inversions. During this sequence, your head will have been below your hips for quite a while. Take your time coming out of it so that you don't get dizzy or light-headed or risk falling over. If you have any doubts about your ability to do this sequence safely, please talk to your medical doctor. If you have been given permission to practice yoga, consider seeking out a qualified local yoga teacher to help you do this sequence safely once or twice before you try it on your own.

The Summer Solstice

This is the season when the God, the male, or the electric force surges forth in full power. As the height of summer, this is the perfect time to nurture the seeds planted in our mental gardens during the spring. It's also an excellent time to weed out those things that impair the growth of those seeds. Traditionally, celebrations during this time of year include bonfires meant to purify and protect.

A Yoga Sequence for the Summer Solstice

The God and the electric forces of the universe have the most power at the summer solstice. Witches can take advantage of this power surge through the various summer rites in order to project the negative or dangerous away and to protect themselves from harm. However, this time of year is also wonderful for working for health, strength, and vitality, as it is deeply connected with the energies of the sun. As with the Beltane yoga sequence, it might be a nice idea to take this yoga practice outside into the sun. Anytime between dawn and high noon is a great time to do this particular practice, provided you are healthy enough to be outside in the sun.

Like the sun in summer, backbends in yoga are warming for the body and the mind. By opening the heart to the sky, we take some of the solar energies into ourselves. When it comes to backbends though, more is not always better. Be gentle with yourself, and listen to your body.

1. Start by lying prone, flat on your stomach.

2. Place the palms of your hands flat on the ground, directly under your shoulders. Hug the elbows into your body as you press the tops of your feet, your thighs, and your hips firmly into the ground beneath you. As you inhale, lift the chest up off the ground by straightening the arms. Only go high enough to lift up your chest and abdomen. Keep your hips pressed firmly against the ground. Firm the shoulder blades against the spine, and pull the shoulders down and away from your ears. You are now in cobra pose (bhujangasana). Hold the pose for roughly ten breaths. Then on your next exhale, lower yourself back to the starting position, lying prone on your stomach.

3. If your arms aren't already down by your waist, place them next to your torso with the palms facing up toward the sky. Allow your forehead to rest against the floor. Turn your big toes toward each other, which will slightly rotate your thighs. Then press your pelvis firmly against the ground. On an exhalation, lift your head, upper torso, arms, and legs up off the floor. Raise your arms until they are parallel to the floor. Breathe. Stay in the pose for roughly fifteen seconds, then on another exhalation, lower your body back down to the ground. Repeat one or two more times.

4. Gently make your way onto your back, lying flat on the ground again, this time with your face up toward the sky. Take a moment and feel the sun on your skin. Bend your knees and place your feet flat on the floor. They should be about mat or hip distance apart and pulled in as close to your sit bones as possible. Keep your thighs and feet parallel to each other throughout the entire exercise. You will also want to make sure that your knees are stacked directly over your ankles. Exhale and push your pelvis up toward the sky. Squeeze the glutes and pull the belly button into the spine. Ideally, you want to raise your thighs up until they are parallel with the ground. Some people will clasp their hands together beneath their glutes, but if your shoulders are not flexible enough for this, it is completely okay to rest your hands by your

sides with the palms flat on the ground. Breathe in the sun's rays as you hold this posture as you rest in a glute bridge (setu bandha sarvangasana). Visualize your subtle body being charged with the God's vitality. Feel yourself growing stronger and more powerful with each breath you take. As you exhale, empty your mind and just feel the heat of the sun warming your body up. Take between seven and ten breaths before you lower your glutes back down to the ground on an exhale.

5. Lie flat on your back again. With an exhale, bring your knees up to your chest. Some people will find this intense enough. If so, simply hug your knees and press your lower back into the ground beneath you. If this is easy for you, however, grip the outsides of your feet with your hands as you inhale. Don't allow your shoulders or head to come up off the ground. Keep your entire back pressed firmly into the earth. Open your knees slightly wider than your torso, bringing them up toward your armpits. Now position each ankle directly over your knee and point the soles of your feet up to the sky. Flex through the heels and press up into the palms of your hands as your hands push down on the soles of the feet. In either version of this posture, you can rock side to side or just relax as you continue to breathe in the healing, vitalizing rays from the sun.

6. When you feel fully charged with the solar energy, exhale and release hold of your knees or feet and lower your legs back down to the ground. Allow your feet to fall open to the sides so that the outside of the foot comes closer to the ground. Place your arms by your side with your palms facing up toward the sky. Let go of your control of the breath. Let it return to its natural rhythm, and simply bathe in the sunlight until you are ready.

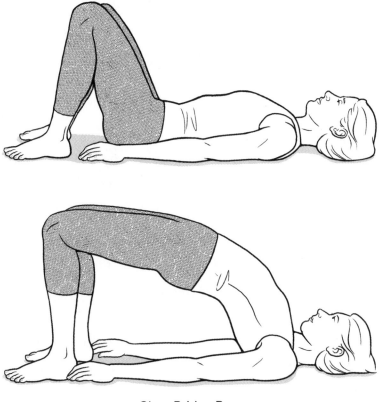

Glute Bridge Pose

This is a time when vitality surges forth in abundance, and we can use it to heal ourselves and revitalize our own energies. All that needs to be done is for the witch to get in sympathy with the solar energies.

Lammas

Lammas is a rite dedicated to the Great Mother, and the abundance of the harvest serves as a symbol of her fertility (and also the fertility available to us in our own lives at the time). It is the natural response to the activities of midsummer, where you nurtured the things you desired to grow in your life and weeded out the things that no longer served you. Some of the things you nurtured are now a boon to you; rejoice in them.

A Yoga Sequence for Lammas

The first harvest is a joyful time of abundance. It's when the Great Mother pours forth all of her bounty for her children. In yoga, this same abundant, joyful, energized feeling can be achieved through the pranayama technique called *breath of joy.*

As with the other poses, you want to use this practice to formulate an intention in your mind. While practicing the breath of joy, hold your Lammas intention firmly in your mind and focus on it coming to pass. Think about the things in your life that you have to be happy about. Think about that which you would still like to see flourish in the coming season. Keep your thoughts upbeat and happy, and focus on manifesting abundance into your life.

1. Stand up straight with your tailbone tucked, your chest lifted, and your shoulders pulled down away from your ears.

2. Inhale, lifting your arms up before you. Then lower your arms back down along that same trajectory on the exhale.

3. Inhale again, lifting your arms out to the side at shoulder height and lower them back down by your sides on the exhale.

4. Inhale one more time, raising your arms in the same way you did in step 2 BUT this time go all the way up above your head, reaching for the sky.

5. Exhale all the air out of your lungs, pulling your belly button into your spine as you hinge at your hips into a forward fold, letting your arms hang down in front of you, like a rag doll. As you fold, breathe out the word *ha!*

6. Repeat as many times as you like. Generally, most yoga teachers stop between three and five rounds.

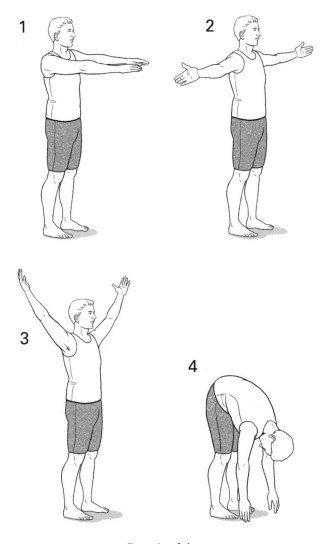

Breath of Joy

Though this is a simple exercise, many people are visual and need to see it done before they practice it themselves. Fortunately, this is a common pranayama technique, and there are countless videos on the internet about how to do this right. Once you see it done once, you'll be good to go.

The Autumnal Equinox

This sabbat takes on the quality of discernment and judgment as its central themes. Like Lammas, this is another harvest ritual, but, unlike Lammas, it takes the masculine current. Saturn, Father Time as well as the Harvest Lord, represents the quintessential energy of this sabbat best. This is the moment where you reap what you've sown. It's the point in the year when you take stock of the mental garden you've been tending over the past year, and you assess what actions have produced fruit and which have left your fields barren, so to speak. Then you adjust your plans accordingly.

A Yoga Sequence for the Autumnal Equinox

We have a tendency to think of yoga as exercise, but sometimes it's more a way of life than a particular set of movements or activities. There is a yoga pose that will help you align with the Saturnine energies of this season. It's called *virasana*, which translates as *hero pose*.

Like the metaphorical bolt of lighting that strikes us with inspiration, this pose produces results very quickly in one who uses it to meditate. While you sit in quiet reflection in this pose, think about your autumnal equinox intention. Look back over the course of the year, and account for your successes and places where you "missed the mark," so to speak. What did you do right? What could you have done better? What seeds bore fruit, and which ones withered on the vine? What did you nurture during the midsummer rite that has grown out of control? What did you weed out at midsummer that you should have left alone? Then, think about where you go from here. Is there a place where you can put your energy that will ensure a bountiful success in the coming months, as we move forward into winter?

1. Kneel upon the floor. If you need it, consider doing this pose on a mat, a blanket, or a large pillow to take some pressure off your knees. If you're really concerned about form and the health of your knees, consider taking a yoga class and asking the teacher for help with an alternative for this pose. If you have had knee surgery, consider seeking the help of a doctor or other qualified medical professional to gain guidance.

2. Place the knees and ankles together with the tops of your feet placed flat against the mat.

3. Sit back on your legs so that your buttocks touch your heels.

4. Place your hands on your thighs, palms facing down.

5. Now close your eyes and breathe deeply into your belly, filling it up like a balloon on the inhale. As you exhale, pull your belly button in close against your spine. Continue this breath for five to ten minutes.

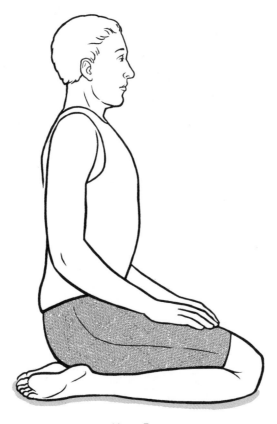

Hero Pose

Start this process roughly two weeks before your autumnal equinox rite. Ideally, you would perform this meditation at dusk (or twilight), that liminal point between day and night. Start your practice taking stock of your year to date. As the fortnight progresses and you get closer to your ritual, zero in on that pivotal point of change, the one spot that, if you were to place your concentration there, would shift everything in your favor. Ask yourself, "How would my life be better if this were different?" Then, after you receive your answer to that question, write down your petition for your autumnal equinox ritual.

———————

The addition of yoga to the various celebrations on the Wheel of the Year helps witches better align with the energies of each season. By engaging the physical body as another resource in their magickal tool kit, witches don't just experience the seasonal energies, they embody them. In this way, a witch's energetic battery gets recharged more fully and psychic powers develop more quickly.

YOGA SEQUENCES FOR
SPECIFIC PURPOSES

This last chapter is really more of an appendix. It is designed to help witches use yoga to improve the quality and effectiveness of their spell work. Whether you're working magick at an Esbat or some other time, these poses will align your energetic bodies and infuse every cell and tissue of your physical body with the energetic signature of your particular intention.

For example, let's say that you want to work a glamour spell at the next full moon. During the waxing phase of the moon leading up to that ritual, you could decide to do the sequence for beauty detailed in this chapter, and, by practicing it, you would "program" your energetic and physical bodies to be in sympathy with that intention. By holding that intention and allowing your mind to concentrate upon achieving that beautiful state over an extended period of time, you stand a better chance of having your magick be successful in this regard.

This theory works just the same with any intention you might choose to pair up with one of these sequences. Some of the sequences below are meant to be paired with the cycles of the moon—some requiring a new, waxing, full, or waning moon, respectively. Some of the sequences can be done as one-offs, whereas other sequences can be done whenever and wherever the witch has need of them. If there is a specific time that is needed for the effectiveness of a sequence, it is given in the directions of that section. If timing is not listed, the sequence can be equally as effective at any time.

Sequence for Developing Personal Power

Fear, uncertainty, and other forms of stress deprive us of our personal power. Left to go on long enough, these factors can actually begin to weaken the immune system. Though we can take measures to minimize stress—we can pick our battles, so to speak; do yoga; practice some other "energetic art"; meditate—we cannot completely eliminate stress from daily life. A certain amount of stress is inevitable. However, we do not have to become overwhelmed by it.

During periods of great stress, this sequence will help, but don't think of this as just reducing your stress levels. It does so much more. Like the sabbats themselves, this brief practice can actually recharge you and raise your energy levels back up. That's because it is specifically designed to increase your personal power before a ritual or spell. When you have a ritual or spell to do but you just don't feel up to it or you don't have the motivation, this is the perfect sequence to do to help yourself find the energy to accomplish the task. This sequence can be done before any ritual. The intention doesn't matter. Power is power, and sometimes you just need more of it than you have readily available. Use this routine to generate it.

1. Start in urdhva hastasana (standing pose). Reach your arms up above your head and press the palms of your hands firmly together. For people with tight shoulders, it is enough to merely face the palms toward each other while keeping your arms about shoulder width apart. If your palms are touching, press your pinkies up toward the sky and allow the thumbs to tilt back toward the crown of your head. Gaze up at your thumbs and take fifteen to twenty deep belly breaths, making the inhale and exhale equal in length. As you breathe, visualize the cosmic energy collecting into one fluid stream and pouring down over your thumbs as it showers you in universal power.

2. On your last exhale, sweep the arms out to the side as you hinge at the hips, falling forward into uttanasana (standing forward fold). Allow yourself to hang there, circulating and "metabolizing" the energy that you have just collected from the universe.

3. Inhale and slowly come back up to a neutral standing position.

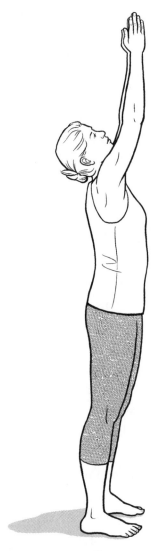

Standing Pose

4. Spread your legs roughly three feet apart (a little wider than hip distance). Turn your feet out to a 45-degree angle so that they face the edges of the mat. Raise your arms to shoulder height and bend your elbows. Once you are in this position, it's time for some minor adjustments. Press the hips forward as you pull the knees backward, creating dynamic tension in your thighs and glutes. Keep your arms active the entire time. Imagine that you are actually holding the sun between your hands. Feel it radiating power down upon you as it pulses in your grip. Keep your head stationary with your chin parallel to the floor during the entire exercise. As you exhale, bend the knees into a squat position. Hold for five to ten seconds. Then, on an inhale, straighten the legs, coming up from a squat, and press the fingertips upward toward the sky, as if you were squeezing or compressing that solar orb, like a beach ball. Repeat this exercise (called *goddess pose* or *utkata konasana*) three to five times, returning your arms and legs to their starting position after each rep. Then go about your magickal working or get on with the rest of your day.

Sequence for Health & Healing

Sometimes we allow our personal power to drain so much that we begin to experience actual physical illness. Our initial dis-ease regarding the normal everyday fears, anxieties, and other stresses turns to disease within the body, and it impacts the body. At these times, it's not merely enough to replenish your personal power stores. More proactive measures must be taken.

This sequence can help in those moments, but it can also be done before your stressors and dis-ease become physical disease. It is not limited to moon phase, time of day, or anything else. We always need health, and the good news is that through exercises like yoga and practices like witchcraft, it is always available to us. This traditional pranayama technique actually heals by cleaning and purifying the physical and energetic systems. It can be done for yourself anytime that you have need of it. Alternatively, it can be done before you go into a ritual or spell to heal someone else. Like attracts like. By imbuing your own physical and subtle bodies with the energy of health, you are better able to pass on healing to others.

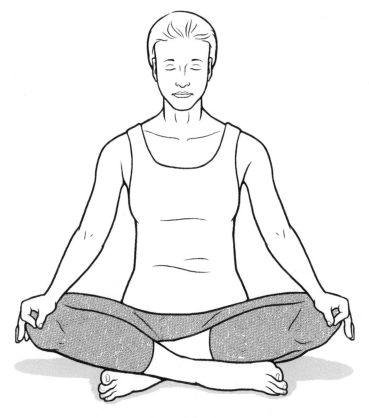

Seated Pose

1. Sit in a simple seated position on the floor with your legs crossed in front of you and rest the backs of your hands on your thighs or your knees.

2. Curl your middle and ring fingers in to touch the tips of your thumbs on each hand. This is called *mrigi mudra* (deer mudra), which is known to boost the immune system, boost antioxidant levels, and calm the mind.

3. Focus your mind on your throat chakra, and see it light up an electric blue, radiating its purifying light out into your head and chest.

4. Gently close your right nostril with your thumb while keeping your hand in the mudra position. (This may take a bit of practice to manipulate, but you'll get the hang of it very quickly.)

5. Inhale through your left nostril. Then close the left nostril with the pinkie finger.

6. Open the right nostril by releasing your thumb, and exhale through that nostril.

7. Keep the right nostril open, and, this time, inhale through it before closing it off again.

8. Open the left nostril, and exhale through it.

You can continue to practice this simple pranayama technique as long as you can retain your visualization of the electric blue orb radiating purifying, healing energy out through your throat. It sometimes helps to see the etheric substance in the air light up a particular color. If you choose to add the color visualization to the inhalation, see the energy entering your nostrils as radiant, healing blue light. When you lose that visualization of the radiant, healing blue orb, you have purified as much as your energetic systems can handle in that particular practice session.

Sequence for Balance

This sequence helps witches balance their heads with their hearts and use the root to ground and stabilize. It focuses on poses and visualizations meant to engage the crown, heart, and root chakras in a balanced way and provide greater mental and emotional clarity. This sequence is useful in aligning with your true will and knowing "what thou wilt" as opposed to what you only think you want. It is also useful for any rituals that require witches to balance the pillars of severity and mercy within themselves. Technically, this sequence could also be done for any ritual where you need to clarify your intention or align with your Higher Self, your true purpose, and so on. If you have lost direction in life, this sequence can help you get back on track. If you have a sabbat ritual to do but you're not in the right headspace for it, this exercise can help get you out there as well. If you have an Esbat or spell to do, but you can't figure out the intention or the proper wording for a particular petition, do this simple sequence. There really is no limit to the wonderful ways that a witch could use this sequence in their magick.

What makes it even better is that something this powerful is so simple. Cat and cow are actually two separate poses, but they are so often paired together that most yoga students in the West think of them as one unified pose. While I only mention the crown, the heart, and the root chakras in this section's introduction, this pose is actually good for nearly every energy center in the upper body. By stimulating the root chakra with the pelvic tucks, it churns the personal power center. Through the undulating motion of the spine, it pulls that power up through the heart chakra and into the head. As it travels through the upper body, the motion strengthens the back and all the muscles of the torso while also massaging all the internal organs. As the head tips back in cow pose, the energy can be directed back toward the crown chakra, bringing about insight and wisdom.

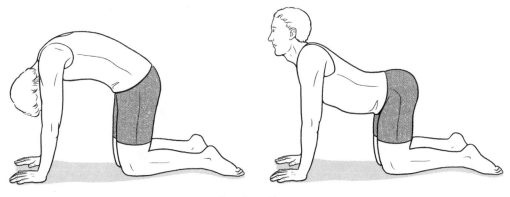

Cat-Cow Pose

1. Start on your hands and knees with your hands directly under your shoulders and your knees positioned under your hips.

2. As you inhale, pull your tailbone up toward the sky and engage your root chakra. (See a light begin to glow in your root, and as you move your body in a wavelike motion, the light travels along your spine to the next chakra in the system.) Drop your belly to the ground, arching your back as you lift your chest up, pulling it forward between your arms. This will open up your heart chakra. See the wave of light pass through your heart as it moves on to

the next chakra in the system. Then lift your chin and gaze up toward the sky, engaging the crown chakra just like the other two.

3. As you begin to exhale, see the wave of light grow in intensity and power as it moves back down your chakra system. Tuck your chin, draw your belly button in close to your spine as you round your shoulder blades up to the sky, and tuck your tailbone.

4. Repeat this process, visualizing the light traveling along your spine and through each of your chakras in turn as you inhale into cow and exhale into cat.

Sequence for Inner Peace

All yoga produces a sense of calm and peace in anyone who practices the asanas long enough and consistently enough. Even the most vigorous and energetic poses leave you feeling euphoric after your practice is over and you step off the mat. However, some of the most effective poses for generating inner peace are the most passive. My personal favorite is legs up the wall pose with your eyes closed. This produces such a unique sense of calm that cannot be explained. It can only be experienced.

Before you write this off because of its simplicity, consider that this pose is a passive posture that is designed specifically to get you ready for a shoulder stand. By embracing the simplicity of this pose, you may actually be able to do something quite dramatic over time. However, for the purposes of our own inner peace, the passive pose is enough. Use it whenever your magickal working leans more toward the meditative methods of raising power. It's also really wonderful as a method for grounding and centering, as you are completely supported by the earth beneath you and the wall. To do it, follow these instructions:

1. Sit at a right angle to the wall with your shoulder and hip bones placed firmly against the wall. (It doesn't matter which side. For the sake of simplicity, I'll describe this for right-handed people. If you are left-handed and you prefer to do it that way, please substitute "left hand" wherever I say "right hand.")

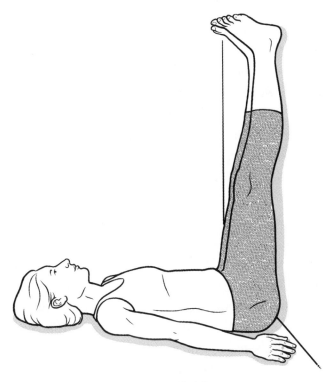

Legs up the Wall Pose

2. Exhale, and in one swift motion, adjust yourself so that you swing your legs up the wall as you bring your back, shoulders, and head onto the ground. How close your glutes are to the wall depends on your body mechanics. If you're taller, you may find that you want a bit of distance from the wall and your bum. If you're shorter, you may find that you are practically pressing your bum against the wall. Do what feels comfortable for your body here.

3. Elongate your neck by pushing your crown chakra toward the opposite wall.

4. Now relax and fall into the ground. Close your eyes, and allow yourself to breathe naturally. Maintain this posture for anywhere from five to thirty minutes or until you have achieved the calm peaceful state that you desire.

Sequence for Confidence

Sometimes we just need a boost of self-esteem. Maybe you have a job interview. Perhaps you're about to give a big speech that is important to your career. Even family and friends can require more of us than we are comfortable giving. This sequence of poses helps the witch generate personal power in the solar plexus and raise it up into the crown chakra and outward. It creates an aura of confidence to help the witch get through the current challenge.

This sequence is good to do before any solar ritual. It's also useful in spells that deal with prosperity, glory, or any other form of success working. Personal growth, accomplishment, charisma—anything where your best qualities need to shine forth, this is the sequence to help you achieve that aim!

During these exercises, visualize your solar plexus becoming engaged. If you are clairvoyant, see it lighting up a brilliant golden color. If you're clairsentient, feel it whirling or pulsating in your abdomen. As you move through these exercises, feel the energy building until you relax into your savasana at the end and visualize that energy moving upward through the rest of your system until you are so filled with energy that it radiates out through the crown chakra.

1. Start by lying down on your back with your ankles, knees, and thighs touching. As you inhale, lift the legs up so that the heels point up to the sky. Do not rush the lift. Allow it to be slow and gentle, and take up the full extent of the inhalation. Pause the breath for a moment at the top, then lower the legs on the exhale, being mindful of all the same measures of control on the descent (i.e., do not let gravity do your work for you). This is a common lower ab exercise for a reason. It's wonderful for both the sacral and the solar plexus chakras as well as the physical muscles of the abdomen. Repeat this exercise for five to ten breaths.

2. On the last round, when you are ready to lower your legs, bend the knees and lower them down together toward the right side of your body. Allow the right knee to touch the floor and extend your arms out beside you at shoulder height for revolved abdomen pose (jathara parivartanasana). Hold this pose for ten to fifteen breaths.

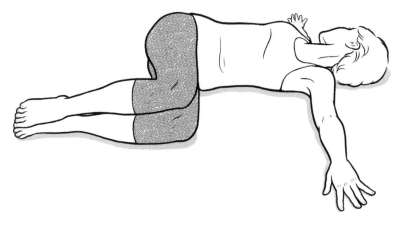

Windshield Wiper Pose

3. Inhale the knees back up to center.

4. Exhale the knees down to the left side for the same number of breaths.

5. Extend your feet out along the ground. Allow your toes to fall open to the side as you bring your arms down by your sides with your palms facing up. Put your awareness back into the solar plexus chakra where you have built up the energy, and with your active imagination, see that energy rising up out of that chakra and pouring forth into the ones above it until it lights up your crown chakra.

Sequence for Longevity & Beauty

In many Eastern traditions, beauty is merely the by-product of radiant, glowing health. The longer you can maintain a healthy state, the less you'll have to combat decay. This is why beauty and longevity are often linked. It has nothing to do with youth. Longevity is not the ability to maintain youth. It's the ability to prolong health and to keep the body from decaying from stress.

We are all beautiful. Our bodies are works of art. Everyone's smile is able to bring joy to others. Everyone's eyes can sparkle when they are overcome with bliss at the sight of a loved one. Beauty is not some commodity that can be bought and sold. It's not something that you have and I do not. Granted, it's something that comes easier to some people than others, but we all have it. All we need is to recognize the essence of beauty within ourselves and project it outward. When our bodies are operating at peak efficiency, they are better able to express outward beauty in all its many forms.

While there are many wonderful poses that keep you vital, none are more effective than meditation. That's because the biggest assault to our health and our natural beauty is stress. Meditation de-stresses us, and it gives us the chance to center ourselves. Fortunately, witches can enhance the beauty they already have with magick. There is also a yoga mudra that will enhance those magickal efforts. It's called the *Venus lock mudra*. As the name suggests, this sequence is useful for any Venusian spells: glamours, attraction spells, love spells, embodying the energy of the Goddess, becoming more likable in general, and so on.

1. Sit in a simple seated position with your legs crossed in front of you and your folded hands in the Venus lock mudra, resting gently in your lap. The Venus lock channels sexual energy and promotes glandular balance. For men, they would interlock their fingers with the pinkie on the left hand serving as the base. The thumb of the left hand touches the webbing between the thumb and the pointer finger on the right hand, and the right-hand thumb gently touches the base of the left-hand thumb. Women traditionally reverse these finger positions.

2. To engage the root chakra and get the primal sexual energies moving, squeeze the pelvic floor muscles as if you were trying to stop the flow of urine. (In the West, we call this action a *kegel*. If that helps you do it correctly, feel free to use that name for it.) By squeezing the pelvic floor in this way during arousal, you are also churning the sexual energies that reside within the sacral chakra at the base of the spine.

3. As you churn the sexual energies within you, concentrate on the action of pumping the root chakra, like a blacksmith's bellows, to heat up your primal procreative energies and stir the kundalini energy within the sacral chakra. Some people find it very easy to do this. For others, it takes time. Be patient with yourself. As the energy surges upward into the other chakras, move your hands up with it as a guide for yourself, and tell yourself that you are "radiantly

beautiful." Don't just say the words, though. Actually see yourself as beautiful. See your skin looking radiant, more youthful, less saggy. See your eyes become more vibrant. See your musculature getting more solid and harder. Embrace all the elements of beauty that are true for you, and fully imagine yourself already in possession of them.

4. When the kundalini energy rises to the final point for each practice session, hold your hands in the Venus lock mudra over that energy center and "program" the kundalini energy to make you appear more beautiful, more glamorous to all who gaze upon you.

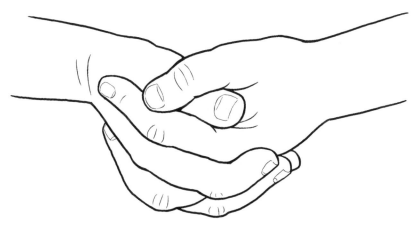

Venus Lock Mudra

Though I talk about this sequence as a glamour for making you more beautiful, it actually has many remarkable health benefits regarding longevity as well. Don't let anyone else tell you that you lack beauty. First and foremost, everyone is beautiful. I know I said it before, but it's worth repeating. We all have qualities that other people see in us and appreciate, even when we do not. However—and here's the cool part—you're also a witch. You can be anything you want to be. If you can't see your own innate beauty, you have glamour and magick that will help you see it or project out the qualities that will make you feel more beautiful. You are not powerless here. Don't let anyone take your power away from you.

In this chapter, I have endeavored to give you sequences for a variety of purposes. However, these are by no means the only sequences for the purposes listed. There are countless yoga poses that would work for any one of the intentions listed. These are not even the only intentions where yoga can be combined with magick. In truth, yoga can be added to any intention that the witch has the willpower to achieve. The sequences and practices in this chapter are really just the beginning. They are only intended to spark the witch's imaginative will and encourage deeper study.

GLOSSARY OF YOGA TERMS

Ajna: Third eye chakra.

Anahata: Heart chakra.

Artha: Sense, goal, purpose, or essence, depending on the translation.

Asana: A physical posture. One of the eight paths of Patanjali's yoga. It was originally ascribed only to meditation postures, but the success of Hatha yoga has transitioned the definition to apply to all physical movements in yoga.

Bhagavad Gita: The oldest yoga book found in the *Mahabharata*. It contains the teaching of karma yoga.

Dharana: Concentration; the sixth limb of Patanjali's eight-limbed yoga.

Dharma: Law, lawfulness, virtue.

Dhyana: Meditation; the seventh limb of Patanjali's eight-limbed yoga.

Ida: One of the three main nadis (or energy channels) in yoga.

Kama: Desire or the appetite toward pleasure, which blocks true bliss.

Kshetram: A focal point connected to a chakra.

Manipura: The Sanskrit word for the solar plexus chakra.

Mantra: A sacred sound or phrase that has a transformative effect on the mind.

Maya: Illusion, but also the deluding or illusive nature of the world around us.

Meru: The spinal column.

Moksha: Release from reincarnation and the cycle of rebirth as a result of karma.

Mudra: A hand or body gesture.

Muladhara: The Sanskrit word for the root chakra.

Nadi: A channel in the subtle bodies through which energy, like prana, flows. According to some Sanskrit texts, there can be as many as seventy-two thousand nadis. However, three nadis stand out above the others. They are sushumna, ida, and pingala.

Niyama: Purity, contentment, austerity, study, and dedication to the Lord. The second limb of Patanjali's eight-limbed yoga.

Patanjali: A sage and compiler of the yoga sutras.

Pingala: One of the three main nadis (or energy channels) in yoga.

Pranayama: Breath control; the fourth limb of Patanjali's eight-limbed yoga.

Pratyahara: Sensory inhibition; the fifth limb of Patanjali's eight-limbed yoga.

Rig Veda: An ancient Indian collection of Vedic hymns.

Sahasrara: The Sanskrit word for the crown chakra.

Samadhi: The ecstatic trance state where the meditator becomes one with the object of meditation.

Samyama: The combined practice of concentration, meditation, and ecstasy.

Sushumna: Often called *the most gracious*, this nadi is seen as "the great river" within the body.

Sutras: An aphoristic statement.

Svadhishthana: The Sanskrit word for the sacral chakra.

Tattvas: A fact or reality that helps connect with the Ultimate Reality or the Absolute.

Upanishads: The concluding scripture in Hinduism.

Vedas: A large body of religious texts in Hinduism.

Vishuddha: The Sanskrit word for the throat chakra.

Vrittis: Mental disturbances that distract us from union. They are correct knowledge, incorrect knowledge, imagination, sleep, and memory.

Vyasa: The legendary author of the *Mahabharata*.

Yama: Ethical rules or guidelines that help yogis live rightly. They are nonviolence, truthfulness, nonstealing, right use of energy, nongreed.

Yoga Sutras: Compiled and authored by Patanjali at least seventeen hundred years ago. The 195 aphorisms are widely regarded as the authoritative text on yoga.

Appendix
BASE POSES

Following is a list of poses that are simple and easy to perform in the privacy of your own home. The types of poses and the specific poses within each category were chosen because they are relatively easy for the beginning yoga student to pick up and do safely and correctly without much instruction or guidance.

Standing Poses

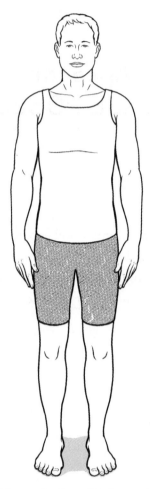

Mountain Pose (Tadasana)

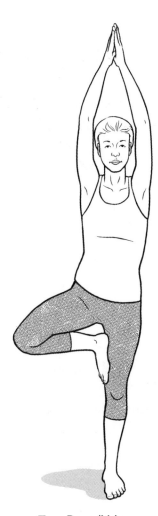

Tree Pose (Vrksasana)

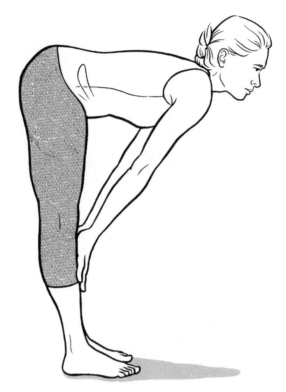

Standing Half Forward Bend Pose (Ardha Uttanasana)

Forward Bends

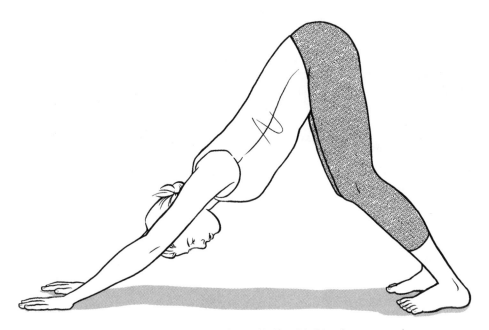

Downward-Facing Dog Pose (Adho Mukha Svanasana)

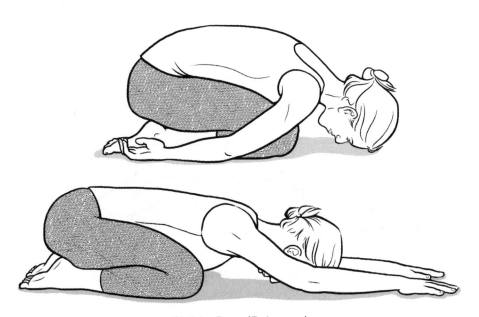

Child's Pose (Balasana)

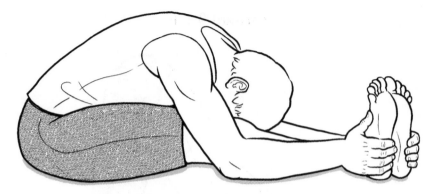

Seated Forward Bend Pose (Paschimottanasana)

Seated Poses

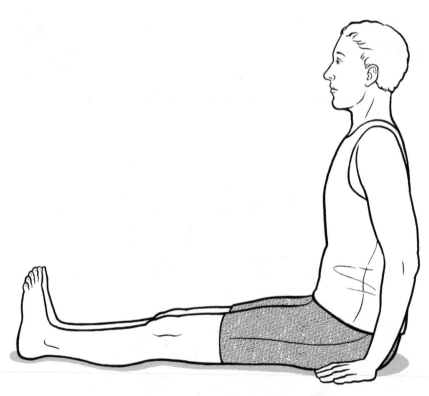

Staff Pose (Dandasana)

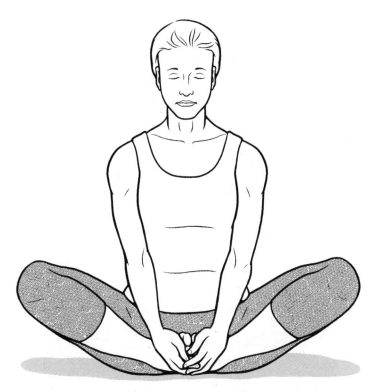

Bound Angle Pose (Baddha Konasana)

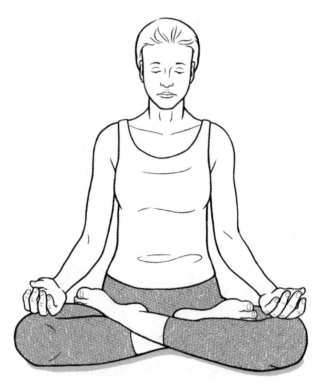

Lotus Pose (Padmasana)

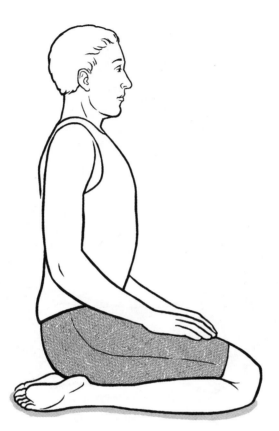

Hero Pose (Virasana)

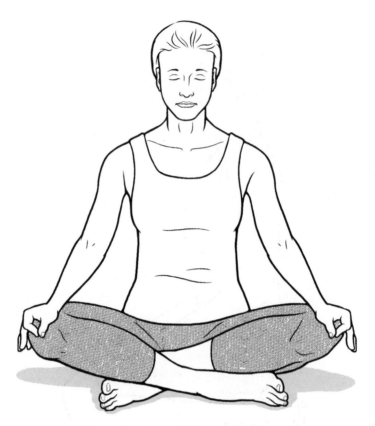

Easy Pose (Sukhasana)

Reclining Poses

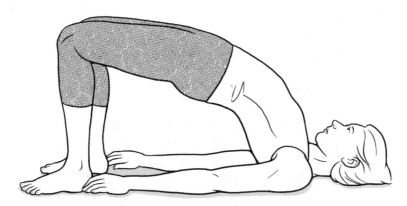

Glute Bridge Pose (Setu Bandha Sarvangasana)

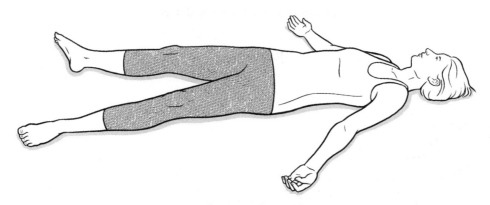

Corpse Pose (Savasana)

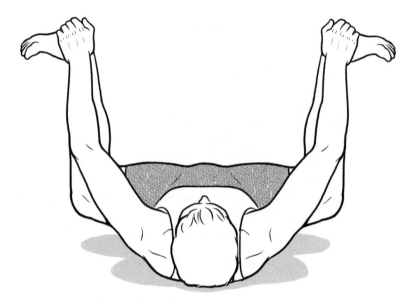

Happy Baby Pose (Ananda Balasana)

Back Bends

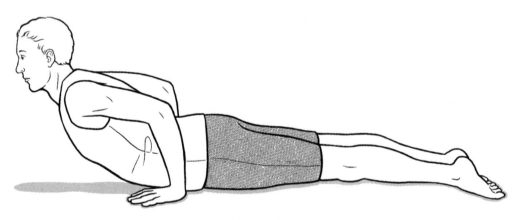

Cobra Pose (Bhujangasana)

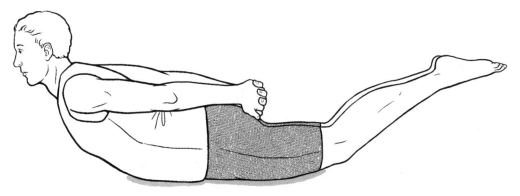

Locust Pose (Salabhasana)

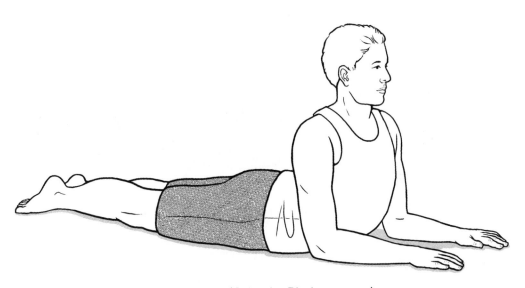

Sphinx Pose (Salamba Bhujangasana)

Core Poses

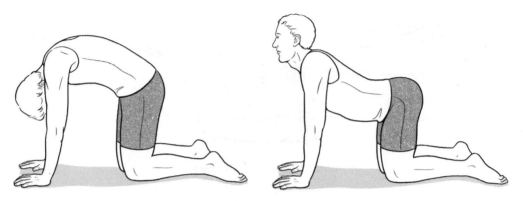

Cat-Cow Pose (Marjaryasana-Bitilasana)

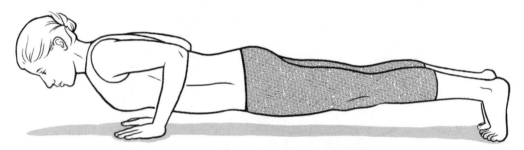

Four-Limbed Staff Pose (Chaturanga Dandasana)

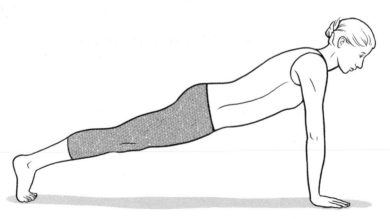

Plank Pose (Utthita Chaturanga Dandasana)

RECOMMENDED
READING LIST

Batchelor, Stephen. *The Awakening of the West: The Encounter of Buddhism and Western Culture*. Vermont: Echo Point Books & Media, 2011.

Blavatsky, H. P. *Isis Unveiled: A Master Key to the Mysteries of Ancient and Modern Science and Theology: Vol I & II*. Independently published, 2019.

Bruce, Robert, and Brian Mercer. *Mastering Astral Projection: 90 Day Guide to Out-of-Body Experience*. Woodbury, MN: Llewellyn Publications, 2004.

Cushman, Lily. *A Little Bit of Mantras: An Introduction to Sacred Sounds*. New York: Sterling Ethos, 2019.

Easwaran, Eknath. *The Upanishads*. 2nd edition. California: Nilgiri Press, 2007.

González-Wippler, Migene. *The Complete Book of Amulets & Talismans*. Woodbury, MN: Llewellyn Publications, 1991.

Hay, Louise L. *You Can Heal Your Life*. United Kingdom: Hay House, 2004.

Maguire, Imelda. *Yoga for a Healthy Body: A Step-By-Step Guide, Combine Exercise & Meditation, 20-Minute Workouts*. New York: Fall River Press, 2005.

Marriott, Susannah. *Total Meditation*. San Diego: Thunder Bay Press, 2004.

McCoy, Edain. *Astral Projection for Beginners: Six Techniques for Traveling to Other Realms*. Woodbury, MN: Llewellyn Publications, 1999.

Singleton, Mark. *Yoga Body: The Origins of Modern Posture Practice*. Oxford: Oxford University Press, 2010.

Van Lysebeth, André. *Yoga Self-Taught*. Translated by Carola Congreve. New York: Harper & Row Publishers, 1968.

Wasserman, Nancy, and James Wasserman. *The Weiser Concise Guide to Yoga for Magick: Build Physical and Mental Strength for Your Practice*. San Francisco: Red Wheel/Weiser, 2007.

Worth, Valerie. *Crone's Book of Charms & Spells*. Woodbury, MN: Llewellyn Publications, 2015.

Yukteswar, Swami Sri. *The Holy Science*. Los Angeles: Self-Realization Fellowship, 1972.

BIBLIOGRAPHY

American Institute of Vedic Studies. "The Meaning of Maya: The Illusion of the World." Accessed July 20, 2020. https://www.vedanet.com/the-meaning -of-maya-the-illusion-of-the-world/.

Aradia, Lady Sable. *The Witch's Eight Paths of Power: A Complete Course in Magick and Witchcraft*. Massachusetts: Weiser Books, 2014.

Auryn, Mat. *Psychic Witch: A Metaphysical Guide to Meditation, Magick & Manifestation*. Woodbury, MN: Llewellyn, 2020.

Avalon, Arthur (Sir John Woodroffe). *The Serpent Power: The Secrets of Tantric and Shakti Yoga*. India: Ganesha & Co. LTD., 1950.

Baker, Ian A. *Tibetan Yoga: Principles and Practices*. Vermont: Inner Traditions, 2019.

Bardon, Franz. *Initiation into Hermetics*. Salt Lake City, UT: Merkur Publishing, Inc., 2001.

BBC Inside Out. "Sybil Leek—The South's White Witch." Accessed June 22, 2020. http://www.bbc.co.uk/insideout/south/series1/sybil-leek-shtml.

Besant, Annie. *The Seven Principles of Man*. London: The Theosophical Publishing Society, 1909.

Blavatsky, H. P. *The Key to Theosophy*. New Zealand: Pantianos Classics, 1889.

Braud, William. "Patañjali Yoga and Siddhis: Their Relevance to Parapsychological Theory and Research." In *Handbook of Indian Psychology*, edited by K. R. Rao, A. C. Paranjpe, and A. K. Dalal, 217–43. New Delhi, India: Cambridge University Press India/Foundation Books, 2008.

California College of Ayurveda. "The Five Elements: Air in Ayurveda." Accessed July 5, 2020. https://www.ayurvedacollege.com/blog/five-elements-air-ayurveda/.

———. "The Five Elements: Earth in Ayurveda." Accessed July 5, 2020. https://www.ayurvedacollege.com/blog/five-elements-earth-ayurveda/.

———. "The Five Elements: Ether in Ayurveda." Accessed July 5, 2020. https://www.ayurvedacollege.com/blog/five-elements-ether-ayurveda/.

———. "The Five Elements: Fire in Ayurveda." Accessed July 5, 2020. https://www.ayurvedacollege.com/blog/five-elements-fire-ayurveda/.

———. "The Five Elements in Ayurvedic Medicine." Accessed July 4, 2020. https://www.ayurvedacollege.com/blog/five-elements-ayurvedic-medicine/.

———. "The Five Elements: Water in Ayurveda." Accessed July 5, 2020. https://www.ayurvedacollege.com/blog/five-elements-water-ayurveda/.

Crowley, Aleister. *Eight Lectures on Yoga*. Las Vegas: New Falcon Publications, 1992.

de Purucker, G. *Golden Precepts of Esotericism*. Pasadena, CA: Theosophical University Press, 1979.

Descartes, René. *Discourse on Method*. Auckland: SMK Books, 2009.

Deslippe, Philip, ed. *The Kybalion: The Definitive Edition*. New York: Jeremy P. Tarcher/Penguin Group (USA), 2009.

Diamond, Debra, ed. *Yoga: The Art of Transformation*. Washington, DC: Smithsonian Books, 2013.

Encyclopedia Britannica. "New Age Movement: Religious Movement." Accessed July 13, 2020. https://www.britannica.com/topic/New-Age-movement.

Gardner, Gerald B. *Witchcraft Today*. New York: Citadel Press, 1970.

Hindu Human Rights Worldwide. "Chakras within the Vedas: Stopping Scholarly Distortion of Vedic Texts." Accessed July 13, 2020. https://www.hinduhuman rights.info/chakras-within-the-vedas-stopping-scholarly-distortion-of-vedic -teachings/.

Iyengar, B. K. S. *Light on the Yoga Sutras of Patanjali*. United Kingdom: HarperCollins UK, 2002.

James, William. *The Principles of Psychology*. Mineola: Dover Publications, 1950.

Kripalu. "The Connection Between Yoga and Ayurveda." Accessed July 15, 2020. https://kripalu.org/resources/connection-between-yoga-and-ayurveda.

Leadbetter, Clayton W., ed. *Aradia or the Gospel of the Witches*. Franklin Lakes, NJ: New Page Books, 2003.

Leek, Sybil. *The Complete Art of Witchcraft: Penetrating the Mystery behind Magic Powers*. New York: Signet, 1971.

Leland, Kurt. "The Rainbow Body: How the Western Chakra System Came to Be." *Quest*, Spring 2017.

Little, Tias. *Yoga of the Subtle Body: A Guide to the Physical and Energetic Anatomy of Yoga*. Boulder, CO: Shambhala Publications, 2016.

Murphy-Hiscock, Arin. *The Way of the Hedge Witch*. Massachusetts: Provenance Press, 2009.

Nhat Hanh, Thich. *Touching Peace: Practicing the Art of Mindful Living*. California: Parallax Press, 2009.

Patanjali. *Patanjali's Yoga Sutras*. Translated by M. A. Rama Prasada. New York: AMS Press, Inc., 1974.

Prabhavananda, Swami. *The Yoga Aphorisms of Patanjali*. Translated by Swami Prabhavananda and Christopher Isherwood. California: The Vedanta Society Of Southern California, 1953.

Randolph, Vance. *Ozark Magic and Folklore*. New York: Dover Publications, 1964.

Sanskrit & Trika Shaivism. "Vyasa Comments on Yoga: Section 1 (Aphorisms 1–13)." Accessed May 13, 2020. https://www.sanskrit-trikashaivism.com/en/vyasa-comments-on-patanjali-yoga-sutras-I-1-13/632#VyaasaI1.

Saraswati, Swami Shankardev. "Purifying the Five Elements of Our Being." Accessed July 20, 2020. https://www.yogajournal.com/teach/purifying-the-five-elements-of-our-being.

Simmons, S. P., and J. C. Simmons. *Measuring Emotional Intelligence.* New York: Summit Publishing Group, 1997.

Stephens, Mark. *Teaching Yoga: Essential Foundations and Techniques.* Berkeley, California: North Atlantic Books, 2010.

Stiles, Mukunda, ed. *Yoga Sutras of Patanjali.* San Francisco: Weiser Books, 2002.

Swami, Purnananda. "Sat-Chakra-Nirupana." Accessed July 23, 2020. http://www.bahaistudies.net/asma/7chakras.pdf.

Tarostar. *The Sacred Pentagraph: A Craft Work in Five Volumes: Books I, II & III: A Craft Application of Wicca as an Occult Lodge System and Craft Coven Organization.* New Orleans: Left Hand Press, 2015.

———. *The Sacred Pentagraph: A Craft Work in Five Volumes: Books IV & V: A Craft Application of Wicca as an Occult Lodge System and Craft Coven Organization.* Cincinnati: Left Hand Press, 2019.

Van Nooten, Barend A., and Gary B. Holland, eds. *Rig Veda: A Metrically Restored Text with an Introduction and Notes.* Cambridge, MA: Department of Sanskrit and Indian Studies, Harvard University: Distributed by Harvard University Press, 1994.

Vanisource. "Lecture BG 01.31—London." Accessed February 24, 2020. https://vanisource.org/w/index.php?title=730724_-_Lecture_BG_01.31_-_London&t=hl#terms=A%E1%B9%87im%C4%81la%E1%B9%87im%C4%81.

Yoga Journal. "A Beginner's Guide to the History of Yoga." Accessed May 13, 2020. https://www.yogajournal.com/yoga-101/the-roots-of-yoga.

———. "Purifying the Five Elements of Our Being." Accessed July 4, 2020. https://www.yogajournal.com/teach/purifying-the-five-elements-of-our-being.

To Write to the Author

If you wish to contact the author or would like more information about this book, please write to the author in care of Llewellyn Worldwide Ltd. and we will forward your request. Both the author and the publisher appreciate hearing from you and learning of your enjoyment of this book and how it has helped you. Llewellyn Worldwide Ltd. cannot guarantee that every letter written to the author can be answered, but all will be forwarded. Please write to:

Casey Giovinco
⁒ Llewellyn Worldwide
2143 Wooddale Drive
Woodbury, MN 55125-2989

Please enclose a self-addressed stamped envelope for reply,
or $1.00 to cover costs. If outside the U.S.A., enclose
an international postal reply coupon.

Many of Llewellyn's authors have websites with additional information and resources. For more information, please visit our website at http://www.llewellyn.com.